~ Praise for *Fight Cancer with a Ketogenic Diet* ~

"Like her website, ketogenic-diet-resource.com, Ellen Davis's book is an absolute treasure trove for anything and everything you could possibly want to know about how and why to implement a ketogenic diet for yourself or a loved one in fighting cancer. She explains complex science in down-to-earth, plain English so you'll feel reassured that while this is the cutting edge of novel therapeutic strategies, it is most certainly rooted in fundamentals of human biochemistry and physiology. Ellen has done cancer patients and their loved ones a huge service. This is a one-of-a-kind resource."

~ Amy B.

"I was continually frustrated in trying to navigate through the overwhelming amount of information out there on low-carb, Atkins, Paleo, and keto diets and trying to tease out the information that applied to me. I wish I had found Ellen's book sooner, because it's all here. This is a valuable resource for anyone working on understanding how to make dietary and lifestyle changes in the face of a cancer diagnosis."

~ Alix H.

"Ellen—thank you so much for this work that you did writing this book. It is quite perfect … It is probably impossible for you to grasp just how helpful you and people like Tom Seyfried are for so many. I am very grateful to you."

~ Janet S.

"The ketogenic cancer diet book is excellent. It enabled me to feel confident in every respect of application, and I am so glad I purchased it. The charts in the appendix have been incredibly helpful, as is the information throughout."

~ Sarah H.

FIGHT CANCER
WITH A
KETOGENIC
DIET

Using a Low-Carb, Fat-Burning Diet
as Metabolic Therapy

THIRD EDITION

ELLEN DAVIS

Gutsy Badger Publishing
CHEYENNE, WYOMING

Ellen Davis, MS
ask.ellen.davis@gmail.com
www.ketogenic-diet-resource.com

All of the information provided in and throughout this Publication is intended solely for general information and should NOT be relied upon for any particular diagnosis, treatment or care. This is not a substitute for medical advice or treatment. This Publication is only for general informational purposes. It is strongly encouraged that individuals and their families consult with qualified medical professionals for treatment and related advice on individual cases before beginning any diet. Decisions relating to the prevention, detection and treatment of all health issues should be made only after discussing the risks and benefits with your health-care provider, taking into account your personal medical history, your current situation and your future health risks and concerns. If you are pregnant, nursing, diabetic, on medication, have a medical condition, or are beginning a health or weight control program, consult your physician before using products or services discussed in this Publication and before making any other dietary changes. The author and publisher cannot guarantee that the information in this Publication is safe and proper for every reader. For this reason, this Publication is sold without warranties or guarantees of any kind, express or implied, and the author and publisher disclaim any liability, loss or damage caused by the contents, either directly or consequentially. Statements made in this Publication have not been evaluated by the U.S. Food and Drug Administration or any other government regulatory body. Products, services and methods discussed in this Publication are not intended to diagnose, treat, cure or prevent any disease. Full legal disclaimer can be found here: http://www.ketogenic-diet-resource.com/legal-disclaimer.html.

Fight Cancer with a Ketogenic Diet / Ellen Davis, Third Edition

ISBN 978-1-9437210-3-0 (Paperback)
ISBN 978-1-9437210-4-7 (Electronic)

To everyone struggling with the harsh reality of a cancer diagnosis and, especially, to my mother, who died of liver cancer at the young age of sixty-three. I wish with all my heart that I had known then what I know now.

"Like a phoenix, they will rise from the ashes of despair and soar."

~ Unknown

Acknowledgments

To Dr. Thomas Seyfried, for your exceptional work and courage in bridging the gaps in the Warburg hypothesis and bringing the idea that cancer is a metabolic disease into focus again. I believe your book and your work will revolutionize the treatment of cancer, and, as a result, many more people will be helped and healed. Your participation in the writing of this book is deeply appreciated.

To Dr. Dominic D'Agostino, for your support and guidance. It has enhanced so many aspects of my journey in learning about ketogenic diets. Your willingness to spend your limited free time and to share your expertise in helping me create this book reflects the depth of your generous and caring spirit.

To Miriam Kalamian, for your clinical expertise in the metabolic care of people with cancer. I am grateful for the assistance you have provided in the creation of this book and in answering the many additional questions from readers. You're a kind and thoughtful person, and I deeply value your friendship and guidance. Thank you for your generosity in providing your expert opinion and aid to this effort.

To Dr. Angela Poff, Amy Berger, and Patricia Daly, for taking time out of your day to read this material and give me your edits and suggestions. Your help and support have contributed much to this work. Thank you so much for sharing your experiences and knowledge.

To my partner in life, Clair Schwan, for your detailed editing and excellent suggestions. You have made this book so much better than it would have been. You're a good man, and I appreciate you more every day.

To Travis Christofferson, Andrew Scarborough, Alix Hayden, Amber O'Hearn, Ivor Cummins, Dr. Jeff Gerber, Fred and Alice Ottoboni, Tim Ferriss, and Robb Wolf, thank you for writing and blogging about ketogenic diets for cancer. Your work adds to the evidence that the dietary advice given to those diagnosed with cancer can be improved. You are helping so many others.

And finally, a big thank you to all the people who have written to let me know how much they appreciated the earlier editions of this book. Your suggestions for improvements were appreciated, and I have incorporated many of your ideas and comments in the new editions.

Contents

Foreword

"Cancer growth and progression can be managed by following a whole-body transition from fermentable metabolites, primarily glucose and glutamine, to respiratory metabolites, primarily ketone bodies. This transition will reduce tumor vascularity and inflammation while enhancing tumor-cell death."

~Thomas Seyfried, PhD

Emerging evidence indicates that cancer is primarily a type of mitochondrial metabolic disease. Although the scientific evidence supporting the mitochondrial origin of cancer is strong, many of those working in the academic and pharmaceutical oncology fields cling to the opinion that cancer is primarily a genetic disease. The therapeutic approach to cancer management is different depending on whether cancer is viewed as a metabolic disease or as a genetic disease. Most of the therapies developed to treat cancer today are based on the gene theory and have been toxic, expensive, and largely ineffective in stopping tumor-cell spreading or metastasis, the primary cause of death for most cancer patients. Indeed, it is unclear how many cancer patients die from the disease and how many die from the toxic treatments used to manage the disease.

Therapeutic strategies used for cancer management based on the mitochondrial metabolic origin are designed to deprive tumor cells of fermentable fuels. Tumor cells are less capable than normal cells in producing energy through mitochondrial respiration. Consequently, tumor cells are more dependent than normal cells on the availability of fermentable fuels like glucose and glutamine. As glucose (blood sugar) is an abundant fermentable fuel for many tumor cells, reduction of blood-glucose levels becomes a viable therapeutic strategy for cancer management. The calorie-restricted ketogenic diet (KD-R) is one strategy that can help reduce circulating glucose levels while elevating levels of ketone bodies, a respiratory fuel derived from fat metabolism that tumor cells cannot use effectively for energy. Consequently, a transition of the whole body from carbohydrate metabolism to fat metabolism can help starve tumor cells of a primary fermentable fuel that drives their growth and survival.

Ellen Davis does an excellent job discussing the science behind the ketogenic diet (KD) as a nontoxic cancer therapy in this book. It is important to recognize that the science behind this diet is evolving rapidly, and we can anticipate identification of new mechanisms of action by which the KD-R will be able to help manage cancer.

The KD should always be consumed in restricted amounts, as excessive consumption can cause dyslipidemia and accelerated tumor growth. The KD should, therefore, be viewed as medical food, not simply as a health-promoting diet.

Ms. Davis describes effectively the mild adverse effects of the diet that some people might experience as they transition into therapeutic ketosis, i.e., the state of reduced blood glucose and elevated ketone bodies. She also stresses the importance of having health professionals monitor cancer patients closely as they transition into therapeutic ketosis for disease management. Good record keeping is, therefore, essential when considering the KD-R as a cancer therapy.

Ms. Davis does an excellent job covering all of the "essentials" for cancer patients who would consider the KD as part of their therapy. She also highlights differences between therapeutic ketosis and ketoacidosis, and she distinguishes pathological weight loss due to toxic drugs or cachexia from the therapeutic weight loss seen with the KD. Several health-care professionals familiar with the ketogenic diet are listed in her book, including Miriam Kalamian, Beth Zupec-Kania, and Drs. Dominic D'Agostino, Rainer Klement, and Colin Champ. The information in Ms. Davis' book will be important for both cancer patients and their health-care providers when considering the KD as a complimentary or alternative approach for cancer management.

It is necessary to recognize that the therapeutic response to the KD will not be the same for all cancer types. Some tumor cells appear more dependent on the amino acid "glutamine" than on glucose for growth. The most effective cancer therapies will, therefore, require the targeting of both glucose and glutamine. While the KD-R does a good job in targeting glucose it is less effective in targeting glutamine. We are currently investing therapeutic strategies that can simultaneously target both glucose and glutamine for cancer management. Ketogenic diets will play a key role in the development of diet/drug cocktails for the eventual nontoxic resolution of cancer. Hence, Ellen Davis's book goes far in providing a valuable resource for managing cancer through metabolic therapy.

Thomas N. Seyfried, professor, Boston College
Author, *Cancer as a Metabolic Disease: On the Origin, Management, and Prevention of Cancer*

Introduction

Hello and thank you for your interest in this book. My name is Ellen Davis, and I am the author of Ketogenic Diet Resource, a website that showcases how ketogenic diets can be used to reverse many disease conditions. One of the diseases for which the ketogenic diet is an effective treatment is cancer, and this book is a result of my research to answer reader questions about using the diet for cancer treatment. My goal is to provide a resource with answers to those questions and help those affected by cancer utilize a ketogenic diet to manage the disease and better tolerate the chemotherapy and radiation protocols they may face.

Currently, this dietary cancer treatment is being called "metabolic therapy." With his generous permission, I have based some of the information in this book on the work of Dr. Thomas Seyfried. His groundbreaking book *Cancer as a Metabolic Disease: On the Origin, Management, and Prevention of Cancer* is highly recommended. It is jam-packed with information found nowhere else and offers the technical details of Dr. Seyfried's assertion that cancer is not a genetic disease but is, instead, a metabolic disease, which can be treated with diet.

Additional information in this book comes as a result of the work of Miriam Kalamian, an independent nutritionist specializing in the implementation of ketogenic diets for individuals with cancer; Dr. Colin Champ, a radiation oncologist at the University of Pittsburgh; and the research of Dr. Dominic D'Agostino at the University of South Florida–Morsani College of Medicine. Dr. D'Agostino's team has done extensive research on the effect of ketogenic diets as cancer therapy. The results these individuals have seen in working with various patients include improvements in quality of life and a reduction in cancer markers.

The dietary information in this book is also based in part on a book titled *Ketogenic Diets, fifth edition* by John Freeman, MD, Eric Kossoff, MD; Zahava Turner, RD; and James Rubenstein, MD. These individuals are the principals of the Ketogenic Diet Clinic at Johns Hopkins Hospital in Baltimore, Maryland. While their book was written for adults and children with epilepsy, it has dietary information that is equally useful for individuals fighting cancer. Hopefully, someday, there will be similar teams in every major hospital who are trained in implementing ketogenic diets to treat people diagnosed with cancer.

Although I have a master's degree in applied clinical nutrition, I am not a physician, and I recommend that your physician be involved in the application of information in this book. However, I also believe that each individual should have the final say in his or her personal care. This book is intended to provide a way for cancer patients to achieve that personal care through dietary options.

One last thought to keep in mind is that research on the use of a ketogenic diet for cancer treatment is in flux, and experts are still pinning down the details of how and why the diet is so effective. Hence, the information in this book is "cutting edge," with new research papers being published just about every month. And while a ketogenic diet has been shown in multiple animal studies to be an effective tool in fighting cancer, I do not and cannot guarantee that following a ketogenic diet will stop cancer. I can say that the small amount of current human research shows that the ketogenic diet does work to slow disease progression, and it also helps to diminish the unpleasant side effects of chemotherapy and radiation treatments. These results alone can significantly improve the quality of life for people diagnosed with cancer.

I also believe that each day is a new opportunity for a better health outcome. I hope the information in this book will help you achieve that objective.

1

...

Personal Stories

"There's something you must remember... you're braver than you believe and stronger than you seem and smarter than you think."

~ Christopher Robin to Winnie the Pooh
Pooh's Grand Adventure: The Search for Christopher Robin

The stories below are from people who have been diagnosed and treated for cancer, and who subsequently found and implemented a ketogenic diet. These individuals report that the diet enhanced their standard treatment outcomes, and bettered their quality of life and health.

Alix Hayden, Canada

When I was diagnosed in 2012 with a low grade brain tumour (grade II mixed-cell type oligoastrocytoma) at age thirty-seven, I was placed on a watchful waiting program after biopsy. I would have MRI scans every six months and was told to return to normal life. Of course, 'normal' had changed drastically for me. For fifteen years, I'd worked at a metabolic-research company, and the idea that metabolic and nutritional factors have a great deal of influence on health and disease was not new to me. I wanted to do what I could to turn my watchful waiting into active waiting.

I am a natural skeptic, however, and spent time down a few alternative-treatment rabbit holes before I came across research on the ketogenic diet. As I read more, I became convinced that I had finally found something that had credible pre-clinical research behind it, ongoing human clinical trials, and data showing that it held promise to influence metabolic weaknesses in cancer cells. I began the diet in March of 2013 and have remained on it since. I have felt healthier on this diet than I ever have. I was so impressed and excited that I started a blog (www.greymadder.net) about my experiences with my cancer diagnosis and ketogenic diet, believing that more people needed to know about this option, and collected resources I trusted in the hope that others could find answers more quickly than I had.

In the spring of 2015, my MRI showed growth and likely progression in my tumour, and my medical team agreed it was time to intervene. I had already done my research to understand how a ketogenic diet can work together with standard treatments, and I was ready to proceed. In September 2015, I underwent awake craniotomy, which I documented on my blog in vivid color, including my diet and mental preparations. My surgical recovery was complimented by the whole team; I was up and walking the same evening and was released from hospital less than forty-eight hours later. My surgeon commented during surgery that the tumour borders were quite clear, which is one of the effects noted in animal studies on ketogenic diets.

Following surgery, I had six weeks of combined radiation and oral chemotherapy, then six months of chemo cycles. Through my entire course of treatment, I maintained a ketogenic diet, and I believe that it can be credited for my ability to maintain energy levels enough to stay moderately active and for my minimal side effects from treatments. Having completed my chemo cycles a few weeks ago, it is my intention to continue on with this diet in order to aid in recovery, maintain my health, and, hopefully, delay or prevent recurrence. I continue to use blood measurements of ketones and glucose to monitor my diet, as well as supplements I've added over time. My last two post-radiation MRI scans, which have been done at three month intervals since surgery, have been completely clear.

Andrew Scarborough, United Kingdom

I was diagnosed with a malignant brain tumour (anaplastic astrocytoma) after a brain haemorrhage on a train on April 13, 2013, while studying for my MSc in nutritional therapy at the University of Westminster. I had acquired epilepsy as a result of the tumour and brain damage. After an operation to remove most of the tumour, and suffering with several life-threatening grand mal seizures, I became informed by my neurologist that I would need to be on a cocktail of anticonvulsants for life (however long that would be) at very high doses. These drugs were only partially effective and came with numerous unwanted side effects.

A period of depression and hopelessness followed, with me experiencing continued seizure activity and a sense of despair relating to my diagnosis. After abandoning standard treatment for the cancer, I transitioned onto a carefully considered ketogenic diet and was able to come off my medication completely over time, against medical advice from a host of health professionals. To my delight and surprise, my scans were showing signs of improvement after the failure of standard treatment—to the point where I have achieved complete remission. This does not mean cure, but I am more hopeful than I have been.

I express great relief that the invisible disabilities that were once so debilitating are now managed effectively with diet and lifestyle changes. I would not recommend anybody to do this on their own without the right support, so I am excited about Ellen's most recent publication. I feel privileged to be able to contribute my testimony to validate the ketogenic diet as part of a metabolic approach to better manage an array of complex conditions and even general health, if that is the main aim of the reader.

The ketogenic diet has been remarkably liberating for me, against all expectations, and I feel as though I have my life back again. It takes some time, planning, and contemplation, however. With Ellen's passion, expertise, and care in producing this book, I am sure that the whole process will become practical, enjoyable, and encouraging for those who choose to adopt a ketogenic diet into their lifestyle.

Sara Karan, United States

When they told me that I had breast cancer, I was stunned. I really shouldn't have been though, because, statistically, one in two men and one in three women will get cancer in their lifetimes. That process was made scarier because I was diagnosed at the end of December 2012, and both the oncologist that my doctor wanted me to see and my surgeon had scheduled their winter vacations at that same time. (Sometimes you just can't see a blessing in disguise. Had the circumstances been different, I would have been herded into standard and customary treatment a few days after the cancer was confirmed.)

Waiting two or three weeks for their return filled me with panic and dread, so I turned to the Internet and started educating myself on what lay ahead. What were my options? I found out that my cancer, which had a HER2 amplification, was very virulent, and recurrence was the rule not the exception. Even with the addition of Herceptin to the chemotherapy, the results weren't great. Patients can start to see resistance to Herceptin as early as three months after beginning treatments.

I was up all night, night after night, reading study after study, and I became more depressed as I read. Then I stumbled onto an article by Dr. Thomas Seyfried, "Cancer as a Metabolic Disease," and a glimmer of light started to break through. He had a lot of convincing evidence that cancer wasn't a genetic disease but began with damaged mitochondria. I really wanted to implement metabolic therapy for my cancer. But how?

The ketogenic diet seemed impossibly difficult to do and so counter-intuitive to me. It went against everything I had been taught as to what healthy eating was. My doctor was worried that I would give myself a heart attack by eating so much fat; after all, I was on both cholesterol-lowering and triglyceride-lowering drugs.

Then I found Ellen's book, read it cover to cover, and thought to myself, "I can do this." It was a difficult decision at the time not to have surgery, chemo or radiation, but it was made easier by the fact that I knew from my reading that my probable outcome from standard and customary treatment was poor. The ketogenic protocol has allowed me to starve my cancer to sleep, and I am grateful today (three and a half years later) for the results. I also take metabolic drugs like metformin (I am not a diabetic), DCA, and curcumin, which interfere with the various feeding pathways of my cancer. The results, to quote my oncologist, are "amazing."

When I got the results of my last MRI, I called my radiologist to ask why he sent me such a short report. I wanted to know in millimeters what the size of my tumor was. He told me that it had resolved, and he could no longer measure it because all that was left was a distortion. He said that if he hadn't known that I was diagnosed and treated, he would have looked at this and thought, "Nothing to see here." (Author's note: Sara is writing about her experiences on her blog at http://www.kosherketogenic.com/)

2

. . .

Cancer and Ketogenic Diets

Now that we've shared some personal success stories, let's explore some general information on how ketogenic diets work, how cancer cells work, and how a ketogenic diet and various food types can disturb cancer cells and tumor progression. We will also discuss how being in ketosis can improve treatment outcomes for people diagnosed with cancer.

What is a Ketogenic Diet?

In addition to water and micronutrients in the form of vitamins and minerals, our bodies need three main food macronutrients that provide calories or energy to sustain life. These are fat, protein and carbohydrate.

- *Fats and oils* are found in foods such as butter, avocado, cocoa butter, coconut oil, lard, and olive oil. Fats provide about nine calories per gram.

- *Protein* is found in foods such as meat, poultry, fish, and eggs and, to a lesser extent, beans, nuts, and seeds. Protein provides about four calories per gram.

- *Carbohydrates or "carbs"* are found in sweet and starchy foods such as beans, flour, sugar, potatoes, breads, pasta, fruits and vegetables. Carbohydrates provide about four calories per gram.

A ketogenic diet (KD) emphasizes foods rich in natural fats and protein and restricts foods high in carbohydrate. In particular, the ketogenic diet for cancer is higher in fat, moderate in protein, and very low in carbohydrate. It differs from an Atkins-style diet in that protein allowances are lower, and medium-chain fats, such as coconut oil, are emphasized to increase ketone levels.

When carbohydrate containing foods (sugars and starches) are digested, they are broken down into glucose which then enters the bloodstream. High blood glucose can be toxic to the body, so there are metabolic processes that push that sugar into our cells and convert it into energy. Only after this influx of glucose has been metabolized can the body turn to using stored or dietary fat for energy needs.

Reducing carbohydrate intake not only reduces blood-glucose levels, but also the amount of *glycogen* (a form of stored glucose) in the liver. This causes our internal biochemical pathways to switch to metabolizing fat and using the resulting products for energy. These fat-derived substances are called *ketone bodies*, and there are several types. The major ketone bodies we will discuss in this book include *acetoacetate* (AcAc), *beta-hydroxybutyrate* (BOHB) and a third, more volatile molecule called *acetone*. All three have different effects on body systems, but overall, once the body is using ketones as a main fuel source, there are some profound and positive health benefits. Ketogenic diets are great for weight loss and addressing minor health issues such as heartburn and achy joints. However, they are much more powerful than those popular uses would suggest.

In other words, this diet is not a fad. It is a potent regulator of metabolic derangement, and, when formulated and implemented correctly, it can be extremely effective as a cancer therapy. In this book, we will explore the details of this dietary approach and discuss how it works, why it works, and how to implement it.

Cancer Cells Are Sugar Addicts

In 1928, Dr. Otto Warburg, a Nobel Prize–winning physician and biochemist, published a paper in which he proposed the hypothesis that cancer is a metabolic disease.[1] Dr. Warburg showed in his studies that cancer cells exhibited a preference for the utilization of sugar (glucose) as a fuel, even when the oxygen that normal cells use for energy creation was available. During a 1966 Nobel Laureates meeting,[2] he commented:

> *Cancer, above all other diseases, has countless secondary causes. But, even for cancer, there is only one prime cause. Summarized in a few words, the prime cause of cancer is the replacement of the respiration of oxygen in normal body cells by a fermentation of sugar.*

Until recently, Dr. Warburg's hypothesis (known as the Warburg Effect) has been marginalized by the persistent belief in the oncology world that cancer is a genetic disease. However, in his research and book *Cancer as a Metabolic Disease: On the Origin, Management, and Prevention of Cancer*, Dr. Thomas Seyfried proposes the idea that Dr. Warburg was correct, and that cancer is, instead, a metabolic disease.[3] Furthermore, he argues that the genetic markers on which the cancer research community has so fiercely focused are just downstream effects of the defective metabolism of cancer cells. This idea is supported by the failure of the Cancer Genome Atlas Project (CGAP), a multimillion dollar, worldwide effort that was supposed to map the genetic mutation profiles of all types of cancer and find the genes that could be targeted for drug-based cures. Instead, the CGAP found that there are literally millions of random genetic mutations associated with individual cancers, and there were no overall, defining patterns in those mutations.

The story of the Cancer Genome Atlas Project and the apparent failure of the genetic theory of cancer are explored in detail in Travis Christofferson's excellent book *Tripping Over the Truth: The Return of the Metabolic Theory of Cancer Illuminates a New and Hopeful Path to a Cure*. Mr. Christofferson does an excellent job of elucidating the reasons why oncology research funding should shift focus from genetic causes towards metabolic treatments for cancer.

Cancer's Metabolic Problem

In real terms, what does it mean to say that cancer is a metabolic disease? Metabolic diseases are conditions in which the metabolism, or the making of energy from the food we eat, is broken or abnormal in some way. Normal body cells are able to create energy by using the food we eat and the oxygen we inhale to complete normal cellular "respiration" and make ATP (adenosine triphosphate), our main cellular energy source. While some energy production happens in the main cell body or cytoplasm, cells make most of their energy in *mitochondria*, tiny organelles known as the "powerhouses" of the cell.

There are two primary types of food-based fuel that our cells can use to produce energy. The first cellular fuel is *glucose*, which is commonly known as blood sugar. Glucose is a product of the starches and sugars (carbohydrates) in our diet, and it is converted into energy in our cells via a process called *glycolysis*. In normal cells, glycolysis is an initial metabolic pathway in the cytoplasm that provides substrate molecules to the mitochondria so that the more effective "oxygen dependent" cellular respiration can be completed.

The second type of cellular fuel comes from *fatty acids*. There are various kinds of fatty acids, and they come from the fats we eat or from the metabolism of stored fat in our fat cells. When blood glucose is low, fatty acids can be broken down by the liver into products called ketone bodies or ketones. Ketones can be used by the mitochondria of most cells to produce energy. The process of creating ketones in the liver is called ketogenesis, and the metabolic state that favors using ketones as the primary source of energy is called *nutritional ketosis*.

This is where the ketogenic diet comes into the cancer-fighting picture. Most normal cells can use either glucose or ketone bodies as a fuel source. Ketones allow normal cells to be metabolically flexible, so to speak, because when blood glucose is low, ketones can be used as an alternate fuel source. Even the brain and nerve cells, which are heavily dependent on glucose, can utilize ketone bodies for fuel. This ability of most normal cells to use ketones (when glucose is unavailable) indicates that their mitochondria are healthy and functioning properly.

In contrast, most cancer cells have broken mitochondria and limited metabolic flexibility. Without functioning mitochondrial energy pathways, cancer cells can't utilize oxygen or metabolize ketones, and this lack of flexibility leaves them dependent on glycolysis and other less efficient forms of glucose-based energy production. In fact, rapidly growing cancer cells may burn glucose at rates up to 200 times higher than a normal cell.[4] However, a cancer cell's broken mitochondria, metabolic inflexibility and dependence on glucose is why a ketogenic diet can have a suppressive effect on tumor growth. By lowering glucose and increasing ketone levels in the blood, the ketogenic diet exploits the Achilles heel of cancer cells by choking off glycolytic fuel flow.

Blood Glucose, Insulin and Food

While our normal cells are fuel-flexible and our brain does depend on glucose for part of its energy needs, some cells, such as our red blood cells, are entirely dependent on glucose for survival. So the availability of some blood glucose is crucial for life. Hence, there are several metabolic processes in place to ensure that blood-glucose levels are optimal. One of those metabolic pathways involves *insulin*.

Insulin is the primary hormone involved in the regulation of glucose levels in the body. Insulin is made by cells in the pancreas, mostly in response to a rise in glucose levels that accompanies the digestion of foods containing carbohydrates. Insulin's function is to remove excess glucose from the bloodstream and "push" it into cells where it can be metabolized for cellular energy via glycolysis. This process is dominant until a few hours after a meal. At that point, insulin has completed its job, and blood-glucose levels begin to fall. If blood-sugar levels fall below optimal status, (for instance, if the next meal is skipped or delayed), a different hormone, *glucagon*, calls on the liver to provide glucose to the bloodstream by breaking down stored glycogen. The liver may also produce new glucose from "precursor" molecules in a process called *gluconeogenesis*. Either way, the release of glucagon triggers a rise in blood sugar to support brain function.

How Foods Affect Blood Glucose and Insulin

Blood-glucose and insulin levels are regulated in part by the types and amounts of foods we eat. Upon digestion in the body, each of the three main food macronutrients has a different effect on blood glucose and insulin.

Fats and oils have little to no effect on blood-glucose or insulin levels, while protein has a moderate effect on blood glucose and insulin: the more protein consumed, the greater the effect. In addition, certain amino acids have a pronounced effect on blood glucose and cancer-cell metabolism, and we will discuss this later.

Carbohydrates have the greatest effect on blood glucose and insulin. Our digestive system metabolizes these foods directly into glucose, which then quickly enters the bloodstream. Each time blood glucose surges, the pancreas responds by making insulin and releasing it into the bloodstream. As insulin rises in the bloodstream, more glucose gets pushed into cells.[5] Cancer cells are primed to take advantage of these glucose spikes for growth, so lowering carbohydrate intake, blood sugar and insulin to disrupt that advantage is a priority.

Understanding Food Choices

Most whole foods are a combination of the three macronutrients, usually with one macronutrient being the dominant one. The exception to this rule is in the case of highly processed foods such as doughnuts or French fries. Processed foods are usually high in both fat and carbohydrate, a particularly unnatural combination. Whole foods, on the other hand, have healthier ratios. If a whole food such as an avocado is high in fat, it will most likely be low in protein and carbohydrate. A whole food like steak or chicken breast is mostly protein, moderate in fat and low in carbohydrate. Our food nourishes us in a loose three-way "ratio" and understanding this ratio will help you design meals which will keep blood sugar and insulin low and steady. Here are a few examples of these ratios in real foods:

- Olive oil: olive oil is 100% fat, with 0% carbohydrate and 0% protein.
- Baked potato: a plain white potato is 80% carbohydrate, 10% nondigestible fiber, 10% protein, and 0% fat.
- Chicken breast: a baked chicken breast is 62% protein, 38% fat, and 0% carbohydrate.
- Raw spinach: raw spinach is 30% carbohydrate, 30% nondigestible fiber, and, surprisingly, 40% protein.

The overall target of a ketogenic diet is to maximize fat intake, limit protein to what is needed for "repair and maintenance," and restrict carbohydrate intake. Understanding and managing food ratios will help you determine what foods to eat so that you can successfully implement the diet. When carbohydrate and protein intake are controlled and fat intake is emphasized, circulating blood glucose and insulin will remain low and stable and there will be a corresponding rise in ketone-body production. The metabolic state of nutritional ketosis is defined by elevated blood ketones coupled with low blood sugar and insulin, and this is our goal.

3

. . .

The Scientific Evidence

Is cancer a genetic or a metabolic problem? Mainstream oncology dogma asserts that healthy cells become cancerous because a gene in the nucleus of the cell mutates and causes the cell to act abnormally. But as I mentioned earlier, the Cancer Genome Atlas Project couldn't find an definitive genetic cause for any type of cancer.

In contrast, the metabolic theory of cancer holds that cancer develops in cells that have defective mitochondria and impaired respiration. Many people say the jury is still out, and the oncological world is moving very slowly to consider the new research which supports the metabolic approach. However, it is a fact that Dr. Seyfried has shown that if the nucleus of a tumor cell (containing a defective genetic mutation) is put into a normal cell with healthy mitochondria, that cell does not turn into a cancer cell. But if cytoplasm containing damaged mitochondria is put into a normal cell with a healthy nucleus, that cell begins to change into a cancer cell.[3]

In layman's terms, cancer cells are like zombies. They live despite injuries that would kill normal cells. With broken mitochondria, these abnormal cells should commit suicide (*apoptosis*) as a normal cell would, but they don't. Instead, they find a way to live by ramping up the speed and intensity of glycolysis and producing more lactate, an acidic cellular product which can be recycled to feed the glycolytic pathway. It's the classic vicious circle. The cancer cell's turbo-charged glycolytic pathway feeds itself, and the excess lactate it produces acidifies the tumor microenvironment, which increases inflammation and tumor *angiogenesis* (a process in which the tumor grows more blood vessels to supply itself). While the genetic markers for various cancers are varied and inconsistent, most, if not all tumors have broken mitochondria and all tumors produce lactate. In addition, research has also found that as the production of lactate rises, so does tumor growth and aggression.[6]

These ubiquitous features provide support for the metabolic theory of cancer, which in turn supports the use of a ketogenic diet to treat these metabolic factors.

How Ketogenic Diets Work

The ketogenic diet works on several different levels to fight cancer. As we've discussed, it impairs cancer cell metabolism by restricting glucose and insulin. It also repairs mitochondrial function and energy production, makes tumor cells more vulnerable to oxidative damage and turns on genetic expression that suppresses tumor growth. In short, ketosis and the presence of ketone bodies returns the cellular environment to one which is hostile to cancer cell progression. In this section, we will look at the details on some of these cancer-fighting effects.

Inhibition of Cancer Cell Metabolism

To begin, as we've discussed, staying in a state of nutritional ketosis changes the levels of glucose and ketones in the bloodstream into ratios which are incompatible with cancer-cell metabolism. Reducing carbohydrate intake lowers blood glucose and insulin, and this suppresses glycolysis and increases ketogenesis. When glycolysis is slowed, less lactate is produced, and this makes it more difficult for the cancer cell to fuel itself.

In addition, restricting carbohydrate intake has the same effect on the body as fasting and calorie restriction (CR), as all of these biochemical states increase blood ketone levels while lowering blood sugar and insulin. This is important to mention because there are many more published studies which have looked at the effects of fasting and calorie restriction on cancer. Both fasting and CR has been shown to reduce inflammation, tumor angiogenesis and growth, proliferation rates and distal invasions (the movement of cancer cells from one part of the body to another).[7] The limited studies available on the effects of ketogenic diets on cancer markers are, not surprisingly, getting similar results.

The mechanism for the direct effect of elevated ketones on cancer is still being elucidated, but some studies have also shown that ketone bodies themselves are toxic to cancer cells.[8] I am confident that future research will provide more insight on this.

More Work from Less Oxygen

Studies have also shown that the presence of ketones helps cellular mitochondrial processes run more efficiently. Ketones allow the cell to do more work with the same amount of oxygen. This was discovered in 1945. Several biochemists at the University of Wisconsin were trying to figure out how to make cattle breeding easier and they were testing mediums in which bull sperm could be stored for later use. They discovered that when the ketone BOHB was added to live sperm samples, the sperm exhibited increased activity while decreasing their oxygen consumption.[9] Fifty years later, this same effect was reported by Dr. Richard Veech's team at the National Institutes of Health. They studied rat heart cells saturated with ketones, and found that the ketone perfused cells exhibited a 28% increase in work capacity per unit of oxygen, compared to cells using glucose alone.[10]

Lower Insulin Levels

Lower blood-insulin levels also have indirect effects on cancer progression. As insulin levels drop, the production of other cancer-supporting hormones also falls. These other hormones include TAF (tumor angiogenesis factor) a substance that cancer cells secrete in order to build a blood supply network for themselves under low oxygen conditions,[11] and IGF-1 (insulin growth factor-1) a hormone which increases cell proliferation.[12] More research needs to be done to clarify these downstream effects, but what is clear is that lower blood-insulin levels are correlated with reduced rates of cancer development and progression.[3]

Oxidative Stress

Oxidative stress is a metabolic process in which oxygen-derived and chemically reactive "free-radical" molecules steal particles from neighboring molecules, causing a chain reaction of chemical derangement that results in widespread cell damage.

Cancer cells use large amounts of glucose to help protect themselves from oxidative stress, but when blood-glucose levels are low and ketone levels are high, that protective mechanism is impaired. A slowing rate of glycolysis hinders cancer cell defense mechanisms, which makes them more likely to sustain fatal injuries from free-radical activity. For example, traditional radiation therapy works by increasing free-radical activity around cancer tissue, and studies have shown that being in nutritional ketosis enhances this destructive free-radical effect on tumors.[13] Meanwhile, normal cells gain a protective advantage in a ketotic environment. In fact, a switch to using ketones for energy results in a lower rate of oxidative damage in normal cells because ketones allow the cell to use oxygen more efficiently. So, not only are cancer cells endangered, normal cells sustain less free-radical damage and get a boost toward better health when a ketogenic diet is adopted.[14]

Ketones and HDAC

Our genetic heritage, like most other living things, is housed inside a molecule called DNA (deoxyribonucleic acid). DNA lives in the nucleus of almost every cell in our bodies. The nucleus of a cell is rather small, so the DNA molecules are tightly wound together in a bundle called a *chromosome*. Chromosomes are coated with proteins that allow either the expression or suppression of a gene within the chromosome. These proteins are called *histones*, and they are controlled by other enzymatic molecules that change their chemical structure. For instance, a histone protein molecule can have certain parts called acetyl groups added or removed. This structural change then gives the histone the ability to direct how cells control all sorts of cellular processes.

In some studies, ketone bodies have been shown to act as histone deacetylase inhibitors (HDACi). HDACis are one type of molecule associated with modifying histone structures. In relation to cancer, one result of histone deacetylation is that the expression of a particular tumor suppressor gene becomes dominant. The expression of this gene inhibits factors in the cell which would promote the growth and proliferation of cancer.

HDACi can also allow the expression of genes that turn on apoptosis, the programmed cell death that cancer cells are able to avoid. A paper written by Newman and Verdin, at the Gladstone Institutes and University of California–San Francisco, reviews how the ketone body BOHB acts as a signaling metabolite for the inhibition of several types of HDAC molecules and ties in ketogenesis as the common denominator for why ketogenic diets, fasting, and calorie restriction enhance gene expression and improve metabolic signaling factors that reduce disease risk.[15]

More Practical Evidence for the Metabolic Theory

The general direction of cancer research over the past forty years has been overwhelmingly biased toward genetic factors. Progress toward a cure or even an effective, nontoxic management protocol has been dismal, perhaps as a result of this preoccupation with oncological genetics. Dr. Seyfried and others have argued that cancer is not a genetic disease but is, instead, a metabolic disease that can be addressed with metabolic therapies. Their argument is supported by the well-known medical practice of using glucose-like compounds to find cancer in the body.

Cancers that are most vulnerable to a ketogenic diet are generally those which are easily imaged using FDG-PET scans. FDG stands for ^{18}F-2-fluoro-2-deoxyglucose, a substance which is commonly used to detect cancers in the body. The drug is a metabolically neutral glucose analog (it is used by cells, but can't be broken down completely like normal glucose) to which a radioactive isotope has been added. Since cancer cells have an affinity for glucose (they are "glucose avid"), the injected drug accumulates in these tumors, and the radioactive signal sent can then be easily seen with the PET (positron emission tomography) scan. In general, the higher the uptake of glucose that a particular type of cancer exhibits, the more likely that a blood-sugar-lowering ketogenic diet will put metabolic pressure on it and slow or stop its growth.

However, not all glucose avid cancers can be seen clearly on a PET scan. For example, brain cancers are detected in a different way. Because all brain tissue is glucose avid, using a glucose analog makes it difficult to distinguish brain tumors from normal tissue using a FDG-PET scan. Instead, magnetic resonance imaging (MRI) is used to image brain tumors. The contrast material used in the MRI scan identifies areas with increased blood flow, a characteristic usually exhibited by tumor tissue.

Do Ketogenic Diets Slow or Stop Cancer?

In 1995, Dr. Linda Nebeling and her team at Case Western put two young girls with brain cancer on a ketogenic diet with the idea that restricting dietary intake of carbohydrates would reduce glucose availability to tumors while simultaneously improving nutritional status. The results were striking.[16] In just eight weeks, a FDG-PET scan showed that there was a 21.8% decrease in glucose uptake at the tumor sites of both girls, clearly indicating that a ketogenic diet had the potential to slow cancer progression. In addition, both children showed improvements in function and nutritional status.

In 2012, Dr. Eugene Fine at the Albert Einstein School of Medicine completed a feasibility study in which a ketogenic diet was used as a therapy for ten people with advanced-stage cancers. His results were also promising. The study demonstrated the safety profile of ketogenic therapy and justified moving human trials to the next level. At least five of the individuals were able to achieve severely inhibited insulin levels and high ketone levels, which resulted in disease stabilization or remission, all without adverse side effects. Individuals also reported that being in nutritional ketosis blunted the unpleasant side effects of standard radiation therapy and chemotherapy.[17]

Several other studies have shown that nutritional ketosis helps diminish the side effects[18] and increase the efficacy of more mainstream cancer treatments[19] such as radiation and chemotherapy. They also indicate that ketone bodies are protective of normal cells in part because they help reduce the inflammation caused by mitochondrial oxidative stress.[20] Dr. Thomas Seyfried's team has repeatedly demonstrated[21] that calorie restriction in conjunction with a ketogenic diet can:

- Reduce angiogenesis (development of new blood vessels needed to fuel tumor growth).

- Restore normal apoptosis (cell suicide) in cancer cells.
- Destabilize tumor tissue DNA, causing effects that damage cancer cells.
- Reduce tumor size over time.
- Reduce the levels of insulin and the cancer-promoting hormone insulin-like growth factor 1 (IGF-1).
- Reduce inflammation.[22]

The details of Dr. Seyfried's research are discussed in his book *Cancer as Metabolic Disease* and in a published paper of the same title in the journal *Nutrition and Metabolism*.[23] Additional information can be found in *Ketogenic Diet and Metabolic Therapies*, an Oxford University Press book published in late 2016 and edited by Dr. Susan Masino.[6]

What about Pediatric Cancer Treatment?

For those wondering about the suitability of the ketogenic diet for children with cancer, the short answer is "Yes." Ketogenic diets have been used for almost one hundred years as a treatment for pediatric epilepsy. In many cases, the diet has succeeded where drugs and surgery have failed. And these amazing dietary results are even more beneficial because the patient is not subjected to the toxic side effects associated with drugs nor the damage that accompanies surgery. Dr. Nebeling's study involving children with brain cancer (mentioned above) was an excellent first look at the efficacy of this treatment. In some watch-and-wait medical situations, a ketogenic diet can be used as a "stand alone" therapy.

The Complete Picture

When you view the complete picture, a ketogenic diet has a sort of domino effect on cancer. It lowers average blood-sugar levels, which reduces insulin levels in the blood. Reducing insulin levels effectively inhibits the production of other cancer-promoting downstream factors such as TAF (tumor angiogenesis factor). In addition, higher blood-ketone levels seem to protect normal cells[24] and push cancer cells toward a more normal genetic expression, which means they are more likely to die, as all damaged cells should.[25] To top it all off, low blood-glucose and high blood levels of BOHB inhibit the ability of cancer cells to withstand and repair free-radical damage, and finally, ketones can affect cellular gene expression to suppress cancerous behavior. All of these effects compromise a cancer cell's ability to survive. The protective effect of nutritional ketosis is why calorie restriction, fasting, and ketogenic diets (which produce ketones and mimic fasting without the hunger) have such beneficial effects on human health. In fact, nutritional ketosis and ketone bodies themselves are being studied extensively as a treatment for many metabolic diseases.

A growing number of research papers have been published on ketogenic diets and the anti-inflammatory effect of ketone bodies on conditions such as epilepsy, multiple sclerosis, ALS, Parkinson's disease, Alzheimer's disease, head trauma, type 2 diabetes, cardiovascular disease, autism, migraine headaches, stroke, depression, acne, and, of course, cancer.

In fact, this ability of the body to switch fuel sources from glucose to ketones (i.e., to enter nutritional ketosis) is a crucial adaptation that has most likely permitted our continued survival on planet Earth. Ketone bodies act as a backup system when blood-glucose levels fall as a result of either starvation or carbohydrate restriction. Without this adaptation, the human race, from Paleolithic man to the modern castaway, might have perished during times when food was in short supply.

This is all rather technical, so I'll end this section with the quick summation: to fight cancer metabolically, it is crucial that you lower blood-glucose and insulin levels and increase circulating ketone bodies.

And that is exactly what a ketogenic diet does.

The New Research

The human research evidence is still sparse in 2016, which is less a statement about the effectiveness of the diet and more about how studies are funded and approved. However, it is encouraging to note that there are now several clinical trials being funded through the National Institutes of Health in the United States. These trials are studying the effect of a ketogenic diet on various types of cancer in combination with standard radiation and chemotherapy.

In addition, Dr. Rainer Klement's team at Leopoldina Hospital Schweinfurt in Germany published a recent paper that detailed the cases of six patients who underwent radiation therapy while on self-administered ketogenic diets. The patients' bloodwork, quality of life, and body weight and composition were monitored. There were no adverse side effects from the diet, and patients reported feeling good while on the diet. Tumor regression occurred in five of the patients who had early-stage disease. One subject with more advanced metastatic lung cancer experienced only slight progression during three cycles of chemotherapy combined with the diet. Sadly, this same patient's condition progressed rapidly after ending the diet.[26]

In another paper, published by Dr. Natalie Jansen in Germany, seventy-eight cancer patients treated with a ketogenic diet were followed in a private-practice setting. The paper reported that "a clear trend was observed in patients who adhered strictly to a ketogenic diet, with one patient experiencing a stagnation in tumour progression and others [experiencing] an improvement in their condition."[27]

Animal model research is continuing to show the beneficial effects of the ketogenic diet on various mouse cancer models. A meta-analysis of the current research on the anti-tumor effects of ketogenic diets in mouse models was published in May 2016.[28] The authors found that there is strong evidence for a tumor-growth-delaying effect of ketogenic diets in the mouse populations, which reflects the research results from the work of Dr. D'Agostino and Dr. Seyfried.

And, in a 2016 study, Adrienne Scheck's team at the Barrow Institute built on their previous research showing that a therapeutic ketogenic diet prolongs survival for mice with models of glioma cancers.[29] In testing for the effect of the diet on the immune systems of the mice, Dr. Scheck's team found that the ketogenic diet enhanced the immune system reactions of the mice, which resulted in a stronger response against cancer cells.[30]

Compatible Therapies

A great deal of the current research around ketogenic diets and cancer looks at the effects of the diet in combination with mainstream treatments. There are also various alternative supplements and therapies which work synergistically with a ketogenic diet to interrupt cancer-cell metabolism. The section below explores a few of these complementary therapies and supplements.

Ketone Supplementation

In 2001, Richard Veech and George Cahill, two pioneers in the field of ketone research, published a paper in which they suggested that the clinical applications for achieving the benefits of ketosis might be served with a "synthetic ester or polymers of BOHB taken orally." Six years later, Dr. Dominic D'Agostino at the University of South Florida was asked by the US Office of Naval Research (ONR) to study the problem of oxygen-toxicity-caused seizures in Navy SEAL divers using closed-circuit breathing devices. During his investigation into the metabolic processes involved, Dr. D'Agostino discovered Veech's research along with other papers and learned that high levels of blood ketones could help reduce seizure activity by allowing the brain to handle oxygen toxicity more easily.[31] This set him on a path that has produced some exciting research on exogenous (from outside the body) ketone supplements.

These supplements are synthetic equivalents of natural endogenous ketones. When taken orally, they provide a way to reach a temporary state of ketosis immediately. The applications for ketone supplementation are broad. For example, using a ketone supplement at the start of a ketogenic diet could help minimize symptoms experienced during the two to three weeks it takes to make the metabolic switch to natural nutritional ketosis. More importantly, some research is showing that augmenting natural ketosis with ketone supplements could be beneficial in cases of cancer, epilepsy, brain trauma, and other neurological disorders.

In addition, Dr. D'Agostino has noted that supplementation can have beneficial effects even when natural ketosis has not been achieved. He talks extensively about ketone supplementation in Internet podcasts with Tim Ferriss, author of *The Four Hour Work Week*.

Ketone supplements are becoming popular in the athletic performance arena as well, and this sector of interest is driving many of the retail-product choices. The formulations that Dr. D'Agostino developed have been patented[32] and in 2014, the University of South Florida released licenses for the production of ketone supplements to various private companies. There are now many different types of these supplements on the retail market, and many are marketed toward enhancing athletic performance. Product names include Ketocana, Ketoforce, Keto-OS, and so forth. There are also various MCT and coconut oils and powders. These ketone products are safe, as long as the dosing recommendations are followed. I have tried many of these products, with various results and digestive issues, but all increase blood levels of ketones over the short term.

Dr. D'Agostino refers to ketone supplements as a fourth macronutrient. As such, it's important to note that exogenous ketones contain significant amounts of calories, so using them to advance a weight-loss goal may be counterproductive. In addition, there is a product called "raspberry ketones" on the market, and this is not a product associated with the USF patent.

As of 2016, the ONR and other private organizations and foundations continue to support Dr. D'Agostino's laboratory team as they develop and test metabolic therapies such as ketogenic diets, ketone supplements, and metabolic-based drugs. He and his team have published a wide variety of papers on these topics, which can be found with a search in pubmed.gov.

Hypoxia, Insulin and Hyperbaric Oxygen

Dr. D'Agostino's team members are also exploring another exciting line of research in relation to cancer therapies. Other research has shown that cancer cells thrive in metabolic conditions in which oxygen utilization is low (a condition called hypoxia). They do this, in part, by inducing a gene-signaling pathway called hypoxia-inducible factor 1 alpha (HIF-1α). This pathway allows these malignant cells to maintain adequate energy levels through glycolysis[33] and without oxygen. Research shows that tumor hypoxia and elevations in HIF-1α signaling are indicative of aggressive cancer growth[34] and poor patient outcomes,[35] and this provides support for the evidence that a metabolic environment low in oxygen and high in glucose and insulin can facilitate the growth and spread of cancer cells.[36]

Oxygen is highly reactive molecule, and it is the source of much of the free-radical activity in the body. These oxygen-driven free radicals are collectively called *reactive oxygen species (ROS)* and as their numbers rise, so can injury from oxidative stress. Normal, healthy cells have metabolic processes in place to protect themselves from ROS, but as we learned earlier, cancer cells are dependent upon the presence of great amounts of glucose to avoid oxidative stress damage.

Since oxygen and ketones are toxic to most cancer cells, Dr. D'Agostino's team hypothesized that the combination of a ketogenic diet with *hyperbaric oxygen therapy* (HBOT) would be effective in fighting cancer. During hyperbaric oxygen therapy, cancer patients breathe 100% oxygen at an elevated barometric pressure, and this saturates their bodies (and tumors) with oxygen. Flooding the tumor with oxygen while simultaneously reducing glucose availability with a ketogenic diet, causes an oxidative stress cascade that cancer cells can't neutralize. The combination of low glucose supply and excessive ROS puts tremendous metabolic pressure on cancer cells, and this one-two punch is why HBOT is being explored to help enhance the anti-cancer effects of the ketogenic diet.[37] When administered properly, both the ketogenic diet and HBOT are nontoxic and protect healthy cells while reducing the likelihood of cancer-cell survival.

Dr. Dominic D'Agostino's research has shown that both ketogenic diets and HBOT slow cancer progression independently, but when diseased mice received a combination of a ketogenic diet and HBOT, the effect was synergistic and the animals lived 78% longer than the same mice fed a standard high-carbohydrate diet. And when exogenous ketone supplementation was added as well, the response was even greater: an astounding 103% increase in survival time.[38]

This is a relatively new research area, and much of the published literature on combining ketosis with hyperbaric oxygen therapy comes from the team directed by

Dr. D'Agostino and his colleague Dr. Angela Poff.[39] This published research can also be found with a search on pubmed.gov.

Calorie Restriction

Nutritional ketosis is a powerful tool in the fight against cancer as it helps diminish the side effects and increase the efficacy of mainstream cancer treatments such as radiation and chemotherapy. If a person with cancer is relatively healthy and strong, higher levels of blood ketones and lower blood-sugar levels are more easily achieved by restricting normal caloric intake by about 10%–25%. Dr. Thomas Seyfried is a strong advocate for combining calorie restriction with a ketogenic diet to fight cancer, and the effects of calorie restriction on cancer in animal models are also being studied by Adrienne Scheck at the Barrow Institute.[40] As mentioned earlier, the body of research showing that calorie restriction and fasting can inhibit tumor progression is much more extensive, and a search in Pubmed.gov will yield many papers.[7]

Metformin

The diabetes drug Metformin is prescribed for type 2 diabetics to increase insulin sensitivity. The drug works by reducing the rate of blood-sugar production (gluconeogenesis) from the liver and upregulating other genetic factors which improve insulin use in the body. This lowers blood-sugar and insulin levels, which, in turn, reduces insulin resistance. Not surprisingly, researchers have also noticed that people taking Metformin exhibit lower rates of cancer. There are now a number of clinical trials under way to determine just how Metformin changes metabolic pathways to quell a variety of cancers; so far, it seems that Metformin blocks the action of a particular protein called mTOR, which drives cell-proliferation rates.[41] However, the dosages used in laboratory studies of the drug were much higher than what is normally prescribed for people with diabetes. It remains to be seen if these lower diabetes-treating doses have the same effect on cancers. In addition, there is some evidence that Metformin can deplete vitamin B_{12}, and, for a very few people, it can have the side effect of lactic acidosis. Therefore, the addition of this drug to your regimen should be prescribed and monitored by a physician.

Dichloroacetate (DCA)

Another potential drug being studied for treating cancer is dichloroacetate. This drug affects a cancer cell's ability to fuel itself via glycolysis. The lack of fuel stops cancer cells from proliferating and makes it more likely that they will run out of energy and die via cell suicide (apoptosis).[42] Although DCA is characterized as nontoxic, people participating in clinical studies on DCA have developed some serious side effects after taking this drug. One study was halted because of multiple reports of nerve toxicity and peripheral neuropathy from study subjects.[43] The human studies on this drug are not conclusive, and, although the drug is freely available on the Internet (it has no patent), I would not recommend taking it without the assistance of trained medical personnel. You may do more harm than good.

Modified Citrus Pectin (MCP)

Another supplement that has been shown to have cancer-killing properties is a substance called "modified citrus pectin." There are quite a few studies in pubmed.gov showing that this substance can block cancer cells from proliferating, communicating, and traveling within the body.[44] The evidence indicates that it is safe and nontoxic. In one study, administering MCP had the effect of inducing greater activity of cancer-fighting immune-system cells.[45] The brand that has been recommended to me by various experts is Pecta-Sol-C by EcoNugenics.

Reishi Mushroom Extracts

Research evidence has shown that mushroom extracts can nudge one's immune system into reacting more strongly, and this includes being hostile towards cancer cells. Memorial Sloan Kettering Cancer Center's Integrative Medicine website has this information:

> Reishi mushroom contains complex sugars known as beta-glucans that may stop the growth and prevent spread of cancer cells. When animals were fed beta-glucans, some cells of their immune system became more active. Limited data from clinical studies suggest reishi can strengthen immune response in humans ... In other studies, reishi increased plasma antioxidant capacity and enhanced immune response in advance-stage cancer patients. Its extracts also inhibited 5-alpha reductase, an important enzyme that converts testosterone to dihydrotestosterone and is upregulated in benign prostatic hyperplasia.[46]

Note that Reishi supplementation can also lower blood pressure and reduce blood clotting factors, so if you are taking blood thinners or medications for hypertension, don't use Reishi without checking with your physician.

Who Should NOT Follow a Ketogenic Diet?

The following information is offered to help you and your physician or health-care professional determine if a ketogenic diet is right for you.

Contraindicated Metabolic Conditions

Individuals with the following medical conditions should NOT undertake a ketogenic diet:

- Carnitine deficiency (primary)
- Carnitine palmitoyltransferase (CPT) I or II deficiency
- Carnitine translocase deficiency
- Beta-oxidation defects
- Mitochondrial 3-hydroxy-3-methylglutaryl-CoA synthase (mHMGS) deficiency
- Medium-chain acyl dehydrogenase deficiency (MCAD)
- Long-chain acyl dehydrogenase deficiency (LCAD)
- Short-chain acyl dehydrogenase deficiency (SCAD)
- Long-chain 3-hydroxyacyl-CoA deficiency
- Medium-chain 3-hydroxyacyl-CoA deficiency
- Pyruvate carboxylase deficiency
- Porphyria

(Note that most of these conditions are identified early in life although porphyria can develop at any time.)

Contraindicated Health Conditions

Talk to your doctor about implementing a ketogenic diet if you have any of these conditions:

- History of pancreatitis
- Active gall bladder disease
- Impaired liver function
- Impaired fat digestion
- Poor nutritional status
- Gastric bypass surgery
- Abdominal tumors

- Decreased gastrointestinal motility; this may be in conjunction with conventional cancer treatment and associated drugs
- History of kidney failure
- Pregnancy and lactation

Contraindicated Medications

This is critically important: speak to your prescribing physician before making any changes to your medications. Individuals taking any of the following medications should check with their doctor or a qualified and knowledgeable health provider before beginning a ketogenic diet:

- Anti-seizure medications such as Zonegran (zonisamide), Topamax (topiramate), and Diamox (acetazolamide) can cause acidosis and this effect can be even stronger when used in combination with a ketogenic diet.
- Diuretics, such as Lasix (furosemide), should be monitored, as dosages may need to be titrated downward or discontinued entirely as a ketogenic diet has a pronounced natural diuretic effect on the body.

Note on Steroids

Although the steroid drugs Lupron (leuprolide) and Decadron (dexamethasone) can raise blood glucose, in many cases they are needed to reduce edema and other complications for cancer patients. Dr. Colin Champ has advised that, in these cases, the ketogenic diet is especially beneficial as it helps keep blood glucose down while taking these prescribed drugs.

Chemotherapy or Radiation Treatment

If you are currently undergoing chemotherapy or radiation treatments, it is extremely important that you work with a health-care professional experienced in the implementation of a ketogenic diet for cancer. Chemotherapy drugs and radiation treatments have toxic side effects and can rob the body of vitamins and minerals via their effect on the digestive tract and absorption of food nutrients. Chemotherapy drugs and radiation treatments may also impact the immune system and liver and kidney function, and these factors must be considered when planning an optimal diet. If your current medical team is unable to provide support, check appendix B for help in locating an experienced professional.

4

. . .

Goals and Side Effects

Before implementing the diet, arrangements should be made to have a health-care professional who is knowledgeable about ketogenic diets available to monitor individual progress. I have included some recommended health-care professionals in appendix B. Ketogenic diets are very powerful, metabolically speaking, and a qualified health-care advocate can assist you with your individual medical needs and advise you about drug interactions. *This is especially true if you are taking blood-pressure or blood-sugar lowering medications: you will most likely need to reduce your medication dose within days of starting a ketogenic diet.* Again, I strongly suggest that you consult with your prescribing physician before making any changes to your medication.

The successful implementation of a ketogenic diet has two goals.

The first goal is to reduce circulating blood-glucose and insulin levels and, at the same time, increase ketone levels. Not only do ketone bodies help protect normal cells but high levels of circulating ketones make it possible for an individual to tolerate very low blood-glucose levels, so it's important to reach both goals concurrently. Normally, low blood glucose (hypoglycemia) triggers a hormonal cascade to tell the liver to break down glycogen to increase glucose levels. This results in the uncomfortable symptoms of hypoglycemia. But when ketone levels in the bloodstream are high, the brain can readily adapt to using these as an energy source, which reduces the likelihood of a hypoglycemic reaction. This is metabolic flexibility in action.

Meeting this first goal is based on an effective use of protein restriction, carbohydrate restriction, and, if needed, a restricted caloric intake to minimize "after meal" blood-glucose and insulin spikes that can fuel cancer. The ketogenic diet is an excellent tool for this purpose because high-fat foods and the right amount of protein are satisfying, and elevated ketone levels have the metabolic effect of reducing hunger. To achieve this goal successfully, it is strongly recommended that the patient track food and supplement intake in a food log or journal or use tracking software such as Cronometer.com, Fitday.com, or MyFitnessPal.com.

The second goal is to provide treatment for any side effects associated with the diet. This would include introducing medications and supplements to support dietary goals or changing medications as the diet progresses. This is another reason why a doctor or a qualified nutritionist or dietitian should be involved to monitor progress when the diet is implemented. We will explore the side effects and how to treat them shortly.

Goal #1: Reduce Blood Glucose and Insulin and Increase Ketones

As we've discussed, reducing carbohydrate intake and eating adequate protein have the effect of lowering baseline and after-meal blood-glucose levels. We also discussed the biochemical fact that excess blood glucose results in higher circulating insulin levels. This is a significant point because high levels of insulin interfere with ketone production, and they are associated with higher levels of a hormone called insulin-like growth factor 1 (IGF-1). IGF-1 is a powerful natural activator of cell growth and pro-liferation and a strong inhibitor of programmed cell death (apoptosis), both of which promote cancer progression.

Your task in adhering to a ketogenic diet is to achieve a state of nutritional ketosis by reducing blood-glucose and insulin levels over time, which will, in turn, increase ketone levels. Think of it as "trending toward a lower baseline" for both measurements. The overall goal is to work toward a one-to-one ratio of blood-glucose levels to ketone levels. To help achieve that goal, we can use Dr. Thomas Seyfried's G/K index as explained below.

Dr. Seyfried's G/K Index

In the first edition of this book, specific target ranges for glucose and ketone levels were given based on Dr. Seyfried's research. In response to individual variations in meeting those ranges and additional clinical data gathered since the first publication of this treatment guide, Dr. Seyfried's team at Boston College have developed an alternative method for tracking progress on the diet. It's a "glucose to ketones" measurement called the G/K index.[47] This new method should help individuals track their progress more easily since it does not rely on achieving a specific glucose range but rather on achieving a desirable index that expresses the ratio of glucose levels to ketone levels.

This is a valid measure of progress as it tracks the relationship between these two important metabolic markers in the blood. As glucose levels drop, ketones should go up, and the overall target is to move toward a one-to-one relationship between the two measurements. Dr. Seyfried's team has found that a G/K index of 1.0 or below translates to good progress for most people.

To calculate the G/K index, simply divide a blood-glucose level (in mmol) by a corresponding blood-ketone level (in mmol). Individuals in the United States will need to convert blood-glucose values from mg/dl to mmol first. (This calculation is done by dividing the mg/dl value by 18.0.) Here's an example of the steps in the G/K index calculation:

- A US citizen's blood glucose is 86 mg/dl, and ketones are 3.3 mmol.
- First, divide 86.0 by 18.0 to get the glucose reading in mmol: 86/18 = 4.77 mmol.
- Divide the new mmol glucose reading (4.77) by the blood-ketone reading.
- The result is the G/K index: 4.77/3.3 = 1.45.

A G/K index of 1.45 is good, and as ketones go up, it will move closer to 1.0. In Dr. Eugene Fine's RECHARGE study, patients who had the highest ketone levels compared to their baseline measurement did best in terms of stabilization of cancer growth or partial remission of their disease.

When you first begin the ketogenic diet, reaching a desirable G/K index can take two to three weeks of strict adherence to the diet. In chapter 7, "Customizing Your Diet," we will figure out how much of fat, protein, and carbohydrate you will need to work toward a G/K index of 1.0. In the meantime, the guidelines below are suggested for working toward that goal:

- Your individual daily protein intake is set on a formula of about .8 to 1 gram of protein per kilogram of ideal body weight for your height.
- To quickly get blood sugar down and ketones up, Dr. Seyfried recommends a daily limit of less than twelve grams of net carbohydrate to start the diet. The net carbohydrate count is the total carbohydrate count of the food minus any fiber. We'll discuss this later in more detail.
- The majority of calories should come from fats and oils, preferably natural fats such as butter, coconut oil, olive oil, avocado, beef tallow, and pork fat.
- General dietary parameters are based on determining caloric intake for your ideal body weight. We start with setting protein needs, since the amount of protein each person requires to maintain muscle mass for their ideal body weight doesn't change when calories are set higher or lower. If your ideal weight is 140 pounds (64 kilos), you will always need about sixty-four grams of

protein, whether you eat 1200 or 1800 calories each day. We then take into account the number of carbohydrates allowed and subtract those calories. The balance of the calories are then filled in with fats. We will discuss this process in greater detail in chapter 7.

Notes on Carb, Protein and Caloric Restriction

The key to successful implementation of a ketogenic diet is paying attention not only to the effect of carbohydrate intake but also to protein intake. Carbohydrate intake is set very low at the start of the diet and protein intake is moderate to facilitate higher ketones and lower blood glucose.

In addition, it's important to divide food intake over several meals. Even if the foods eaten are low in carb and protein, eating a large amount of them all at once can result in glucose and insulin spikes. Dr. Seyfried has also found that caloric restriction is an effective component of the success of the ketogenic diet in his animal research and in at least one human case study.

For cancer patients who are underweight or nutritionally compromised, Dr. Colin Champ, a radiation oncologist at the University of Pittsburgh reports that caloric restriction is not recommended. However, he states that mild caloric restriction can offer some benefit for patients who are overweight. For overweight patients, lowering weight maintenance calories 10%–25% (equal to a loss of one to two pounds per week) can be helpful and may improve cancer-treatment outcomes.

Goal #2: Minimize and Treat Possible Side Effects

Since the ketogenic diet is metabolically powerful, it does come with some potential side effects. However, it is unlikely that you or any other person on the diet will experience all of the known side effects. Even so, I like to discuss them because they can be alarming if you learn about them through experience alone. The good news is that these side effects are mostly temporary and resolve themselves as the body adapts to using ketones instead of glucose as the primary fuel. Nevertheless, since they are unpleasant, let's discuss them and review methods for minimizing them. *Give this section your full attention.* Not doing so can result in major discomfort and failure to succeed on this diet.

Side Effect 1: Hypoglycemia (Low Blood Glucose)

As carbohydrate intake is lowered, withdrawal symptoms such as nausea, dizziness, light-headedness, shakiness, heart palpitations, hunger, and headaches may manifest. These are indicative of hypoglycemia. Drinking an ounce of orange juice may help after fifteen minutes or so if the symptoms are intolerable. For most people, the worst of these effects should fade after the first four to seven days of carb restriction as the body will begin to adapt to using ketones for fuel. For some, the hypoglycemia may be intense. To manage the intense reactions, it may help to slow the withdrawal process by reducing carbohydrate levels in stages over several weeks until you can stay below twelve grams without a reaction. As carbohydrate intake is consistently lowered over time, baseline insulin levels will begin to drop as well. And as they do, carbohydrate intake can be reduced further without withdrawal symptoms.

Side Effect 2: Hunger and Cravings

Hunger and cravings are normal and are usually one the most difficult challenges for those new to the diet. However, over time, being "in ketosis" and adapting to this shift in metabolism has a pronounced dampening effect on hunger. It may take several weeks for blood-ketone levels to consistently remain high enough (above 1 to 2 mM) to affect physiological hunger. If hunger is still a problem after two to three weeks on the diet, you may be eating too many carbs or too much protein for your individual needs. Review what you're eating from your food log to be sure that carb and protein intake are low and fat intake is high. This is not to say that psychological cravings will also disappear, but the biochemical drivers will be greatly reduced. Eating one or two tablespoons of coconut oil may increase ketosis and help quell hunger.

Side Effect 3: Weakness, Dizziness and Fatigue

Fatigue, dizziness and feelings of weakness or shakiness can be caused by dehydration and mineral loss, especially low sodium levels. Implementing a ketogenic diet usually causes the body to rid itself of excess water. Reducing carb intake has the effect of depleting glycogen stores and stimulating the kidneys. As glycogen is metabolized, urination increases dramatically and minerals such as potassium, calcium, magnesium and sodium are eliminated through the urine. It is the loss of these minerals that results in fatigue and the symptoms of dehydration: increased thirst, dry mouth, cramping, weakness, irritability, headache, dizziness, palpitations, confusion, sluggishness, and fainting. Replace the minerals and fluids by sipping meat and chicken broth and eating more green leafy vegetables. Also, follow these recommendations on mineral supplements:

- Add magnesium citrate supplements as recommended in appendix A. If there are kidney problems in your medical history, don't take oral magnesium supplements without checking with the physician responsible for the care of these conditions.

- To keep potassium levels up, eat more avocado and green leafy vegetables. You can also use salt substitutes containing not only sodium, but potassium and magnesium. Supplements can also be used, but please check with your physician about blood-pressure-drug interactions before taking potassium supplements, and never take more than 300 mg of potassium citrate in one dose. Too much potassium can stop your heart.

- To keep sodium levels up, don't be afraid to add salt to meals. If you experience weakness or a "woozy" or "unfocused" feeling, I recommend putting one-quarter teaspoon of sea salt in a glass of water and drinking it. The symptoms should get better shortly thereafter if a mineral imbalance is the problem. (However, if you're taking diuretics or have been advised to avoid salt, talk to your doctor before adding salt or potassium.)

Side Effect 4: Constipation

The ketogenic diet is a low fiber, low residue diet, and constipation is a common complaint. In my experience, constipation can be an indication of a magnesium deficiency, and/or dehydration. It is also a common side effect of pain medication. Individuals with slow gastrointestinal (GI) motility (due to drugs or disease) should discuss options to address constipation with their physician.

There are drugs for GI motility, such as Milk of Magnesia as a laxative, MiraLax or Movicol (Polyethylene Glycol 3350) and stool softeners such as Dulcolax. Bulky greens such as Romaine lettuce and sautéed mixed greens can also ease constipation. Fiber bulking products such as psyllium husk powder should not be used if you are currently constipated, but can be used after bowel movements return to normal. (See the Fiber section in chapter 6.) However, individuals with ulcerative colitis, Crohn's disease, or bowel obstruction issues should not use psyllium husk. Talk to your doctor about other options.

Side Effect 5: Muscle Cramps and Dehydration

Muscle cramps are likely a result of water and mineral losses discussed above. Dosages of diuretic drugs may need to be adjusted as ketogenic diets are naturally diuretic. It's important to discuss this first with your prescribing physician before making changes.

Alternatively, follow the recommendations of Drs. Jeff Volek and Stephen Phinney in their book *The Art and Science of Low Carbohydrate Living: An Expert Guide to Making the Life-Saving Benefits of Carbohydrate Restriction Sustainable and Enjoyable*. They recommend taking three slow-release magnesium tablets such as Slow-Mag or Mag 64 for twenty days, and then taking one tablet a day thereafter for muscle cramps.

Note that if you have kidney problems, you should not take oral magnesium supplements without consulting the physician responsible for treating your kidney issues.

Side Effect 6: Mild Acidosis

Although very rare, some people may experience mild metabolic acidosis when implementing a ketogenic diet. If you develop symptoms such as rapid breathing, excessive fatigue, nausea or vomiting, it may be that ketone levels are too high. The main treatment is to drink sixteen to twenty ounces of water and warmed chicken broth which does not have MSG (monosodium glutamate) as an ingredient. (Avoid bouillon cubes.) The broth will provide some potassium and the extra fluid will help dilute ketones in your bloodstream. After taking these first measures, wait for thirty minutes. If symptoms don't get better, sip an ounce of orange juice and wait for twenty minutes. If the symptoms don't subside as this point, contact your health-care professional or go to the emergency room and let them know you suspect metabolic acidosis.

Side Effect 7: Ketone Breath

Excess ketones can be expelled from the body via the lungs and in the urine. The main ketone in breath is acetone, which has a distinctive smell. Ketone breath is described as being "fruity" or "metallic." As your body adapts to using the ketones as fuel, less should be expelled in your breath. Although ketone breath may be unpleasant tasting, we consider it a good indicator that you've achieved the state of nutritional ketosis.

Side Effect 8: Weight Changes

A ketogenic diet lowers blood glucose and insulin and, eventually, caloric intake as hunger subsides. High insulin levels prevent your body from accessing stored body fat and using it for fuel. When insulin levels and calories are lowered, the body is then able to access body fat to use as fuel, and this results in weight loss for most people. If you experience unintended weight loss, eat more calories in the form of natural fats (such as butter, macadamia nuts, and avocados) on a daily basis until the weight loss stops. If this does not help, eat more protein or, as Miriam Kalamian recommends, add a quarter cup of cooked legumes (beans, lentils) to your daily menu. Consuming more medium-chain triglyceride (MCT) oil and coconut oil are not good choices for this issue as Miriam reports they don't seem to help with weight stabilization. If you find it difficult to eat due to gastrointestinal issues or lack of appetite, please partner with a nutritionist or other trained professional who can offer some suggestions.

There's a very serious type of muscle-wasting weight loss experienced by late-stage cancer patients called cancer cachexia. Doctors often mistake weight loss associated with cachexia for the more benign weight loss experienced with a ketogenic diet. They may direct dietitians to suggest that you not lose weight, even if you are overweight. They may even prescribe drinks loaded with carbs to keep weight loss to a minimum. This will work to maintain weight, but it will compromise your goals on the diet as high carb intake will interfere with the lower blood-glucose levels and higher ketone levels you're trying to achieve. In addition, research on the ketogenic diet has shown that being in nutritional ketosis helps reduce the loss of muscle and body weight associated with cachexia.[48]

Side Effect 9: Changes in Blood Pressure

High blood glucose and insulin result in greater glycogen stores and hormonal changes, which cause the body to retain water. For some people, this excess water storage translates into high blood pressure. Once blood-glucose and insulin levels start to drop, the body will burn through glycogen stored in the muscles and liver, and this will cause the kidneys to excrete excess water. Blood pressure should drop as a result. For this reason, a physician should monitor all blood-pressure medication being taken. If you take blood-pressure medication, you may find that you become lightheaded and dizzy after a week on the diet. This is a sign that you may need to reduce your blood-pressure medication.

Side Effect 10: Vitamin and Mineral Deficiencies

Because certain foods and calories may be restricted and drugs can deplete some nutrients, vitamin and mineral supplementations are recommended. A basic multivitamin/multi-mineral supplement that contains the RDA for all vitamins and minerals is a good start. Pay particular attention that the multivitamin contains the baseline for zinc and selenium. Appendix A lists supplement recommendations.

Side Effect 11: Nausea

Many people are not used to eating the amount of fat allowed on a ketogenic diet. Nausea is common after eating a high fat meal or after taking coconut oil or MCT oil. If this happens, try spreading out your fat intake over smaller meals and snacks or consuming some of your daily fats between meals or talk to your doctor about high-lipase digestive enzymes.

Final Note on Side Effects and Broth

Many of these side effects can be managed just by making sure your mineral intake is adequate. Bone and meat broths, as mentioned, are a great way to do this.

About Heart Palpitations or a "Racing" Heart

Some people may experience heart palpitations or a racing heart when starting a ketogenic diet or after having been on one for some time. It's been reported that this is more likely if the person normally has low blood pressure. There are several factors which may be involved in this symptom.

- There may be nutrient deficiencies. This is why a multivitamin containing the RDA for selenium and zinc, plus a magnesium supplement, broth, or mineral water are strongly recommended.
- The affected person may be insulin resistant, and lowering carbohydrate intake can result in transient hypoglycemia. Hypoglycemia can also result from not eating often enough or not eating enough protein and fat. (See Side Effect 1.)
- There may be an electrolyte imbalance, or you may be dehydrated. Making some homemade mineral water and drinking a cup with your morning and evening meal should help if this is the issue. (See Possible Side Effect 3.) In addition, drink plenty of water.

Finally, some people may have "racing" heart reactions to excessive coconut oil or medium-chain triglyceride (MCT) oil consumption. As you add these oils to your diet, start with small amounts and increase over time. Don't rely on coconut or MCT oil for your only fat intake. Be sure to include other fats such as butter, ghee, olive oil, and animal fats as well.

Concerns about Elevated Cholesterol

Many people have trouble on a ketogenic diet plan because they are alarmed about increasing the amount of fat they eat, especially saturated fat. This becomes an issue particularly if total cholesterol goes up while on the diet, and the individual's physician voices concern about higher cholesterol levels.

A physician's concern is understandable. The message that eating fat and choles-terol are harmful has been pounded into the collective American psyche for the last forty years. It's also difficult to unlearn the message that high cholesterol is the cause of heart disease. I understand that these messages have been repeated over and over, but they are both untrue. Dr. Ron Rosedale, an expert on ketogenic diets, writes about this on his website.[49]

The real culprit of atherosclerosis is chronically elevated blood glucose and insulin and the associated inflammatory damage to artery walls. This is why diabetics and those with metabolic syndrome suffer from higher rates of heart disease.

For most people, following a ketogenic diet improves the risk markers for cardio-vascular health. Adhering to a ketogenic diet will lower baseline blood glucose and insulin, which will, in turn, lower inflammation and reduce arterial damage. The higher saturated fat intake associated with the diet also increases HDL cholesterol, and, at the same time, the lower carb intake decreases triglyceride levels. These two factors are the major markers for heart disease.

Ketosis versus Ketoacidosis

Some medical professionals confuse diabetic ketoacidosis, an extreme and dangerous form of ketosis, with the benign nutritional ketosis associated with ketogenic diets and fasting states in the body. The difference between the two conditions depends on whether the body has the ability to make insulin, as insulin regulates ketone production. Benign nutritional ketosis is an insulin regulated process that results in a mild release of fatty acids and a moderate conversion of fatty acids to ketone bodies.

Diabetic ketoacidosis is a condition in which insulin is unavailable, either because the pancreas cannot make it (type 1 Diabetes) or because body cells are insulin resis-tant (type 2 Diabetes). As a result, blood glucose climbs to high levels and excessive quantities of ketones are produced in an unregulated biochemical state. Diabetic keto-acidosis has little in common with nutritional ketosis. DKA is a dangerous medical condition caused by a deficiency of insulin, often in the setting of illness, typically a serious infection. The list below itemizes ketone concentrations in the body to help differentiate between ketosis and ketoacidosis:

- After a meal, ketones may drop to 0.1 mmol/L
- An overnight fast will raise ketones to 0.3 mmol/L
- A state of nutritional ketosis can raise ketones to 1.0 to 8.0 mmol/L. However, it also decreases blood sugar to normal ranges.

- Less than twenty days of fasting will result in ketone levels of less than 10.0 mmol/L and blood sugars of 65–75 mg/dL.
- Diabetic ketoacidosis will raise ketones to very high levels of greater than 10.0–15.0 mmol/L and will also raise blood-glucose levels in excess of 250 mg/dL.

The danger of ketoacidosis is in the high blood sugar and amount of ketone bodies being generated. Ketone bodies are slightly acidic in nature, and, in the absence of insulin, so many are generated at once that they build up in the bloodstream. The sheer volume quickly overwhelms the delicate acid-base buffering system of the blood, and the blood becomes more acidic than normal. It is this acidic condition that is dangerous, not the ketones themselves.

5

...

Benefits and Monitoring Progress

Since we talked about the side effects in the previous chapter, I want to also discuss the benefits associated with a ketogenic diet. They are numerous and affect many different body systems. The details are below.

- *Lower Blood-Sugar (Glucose) and HbA1c Levels:* When carbohydrates are consumed and digested, they cause a sharp increase in blood sugar. This sugar sticks to many body proteins that it touches, including those in red blood cells. This process is called glycation, and it is measured by a blood test called a hemoglobin A1c or HbA1c. HbA1c levels are a strong marker for the overall state of health. Elevated HbA1c results are linked to heart disease, cancer, autoimmune conditions, and many inflammatory diseases.[50] Ketogenic diets lower blood sugar and glycation events and, therefore, HbA1c levels.

- *Improving Insulin Resistance:* Insulin is a hormone secreted by the pancreas to manage blood-sugar levels. One of insulin's jobs is to push blood sugar into cells so it can be used for fuel. Insulin is also a signaling hormone, and it has many downstream effects. When blood levels of insulin are inappropriately elevated over time, the result is insulin resistance, a condition linked to many disease states. When carb intake is restricted, insulin resistance improves. This is one of the most powerful benefits of a ketogenic diet.[51]

- *Decrease in Triglycerides:* Triglycerides are fat molecules that are normally stored in our fat cells. Consuming large amounts of carbohydrates causes a rise in the amount of triglyceride in the bloodstream instead. High blood-triglyceride levels are a major marker for heart disease. The less carbohydrate you eat, the lower your blood triglyceride readings will be, especially if you suffer from conditions such as insulin resistance or metabolic syndrome.[52]

- *Increase in HDL Cholesterol and Better Heart Disease Risks:* Following a keto-genic diet will raise "good" HDL cholesterol in the blood while lowering the "bad" LDL cholesterol, blood triglycerides, and total cholesterol.[53] This positive change improves the ratio of good to bad cholesterol, and, more important, the ratio of triglycerides/HDL. A triglyceride/HDL ratio of 1.0 or less is considered optimal and indicates an extremely low risk of a heart-attack event.[54]

- *For People with Diabetes, Fewer Diabetes Medications and Lower Insulin Doses:* The ketogenic diet is very effective for the prevention and treatment of pre-diabetes and type 1 and type 2 diabetes because it limits dietary carbohydrate and normalizes the amount of sugar or glucose in the blood. This results in a lower need for insulin from either the pancreas[55] or from injections. For persons with type 2 diabetes, the diet improves insulin resistance and subsequently improves blood-glucose control with a significant reduction in medication needs.[56] For persons with type 1 diabetes, insulin requirements are reduced, blood-glu-cose control is improved, and low-blood-sugar episodes (hypoglycemia) are reduced, as shown in a study by a team of Swedish medical researchers in which compliant patients reduced their average blood glucose from 14 mM (250 mg/dL) to 6.4 mM (115 mg/dL).[57] (NOTE: If you take any medication to lower your blood sugar such as Metformin or insulin, you will most likely need to reduce you dosage almost immediately upon starting a ketogenic diet. I strongly suggest that you consult with your prescribing physician before start-ing the diet or making any changes to your medication. See my books *Conquer Type 2 Diabetes with a Ketogenic Diet* and *The Ketogenic Diet for Type 1 Diabetes* for more information.)

- *Lower Blood Pressure:* Ketogenic diets are very effective at reducing the under-lying insulin resistance that elevates blood pressure.[58] Elevated blood-ketone levels relax blood vessels and lower insulin levels allowing the kidneys to release excess salt and water.

- *Lower Levels of Inflammation:* Ketogenic diets exert anti-inflammatory effects by normalizing immune-system activity. Inflammation is a major driver of dis-ease, and it is measured using a high-sensitivity C-reactive protein (hs-CRP) test. Starting a ketogenic diet lowers hs-CRP and other markers of inflamma-tion as shown in a study by Dr. Jeff Volek's team at the University of Connecti-cut. They reported that subjects on a low-carbohydrate diet saw a significant reduction of seven different inflammatory cytokines, evidence that being on a ketogenic diet suppresses immune-system mediated inflammation.[59]

- *Heartburn Relief:* Many people who suffer from gastroesophageal reflux disease (GERD) or other heartburn issues notice improvement in their symptoms after starting a ketogenic diet. One of the major causes of GERD is fermentable carbohydrate consumption and, in particular, gluten grains[60], and these foods are restricted on a ketogenic diet. A study by Dr. Eric Westman's team at the University of North Carolina reported that a low-carbohydrate diet can significantly improve symptoms in obese individuals with GERD.[61]

- *Less Gum and Tooth Disease:* Carbohydrate consumption lowers the pH of your saliva and contributes to tooth decay[62], and, not surprisingly, people with high blood sugar have a higher rate of periodontal disease.[63] Adopting a ketogenic diet improves dental health and reduces tooth decay because it reduces the amount of carbohydrate consumed.

- *Improvement in Mental Health Disorders:* The ketogenic diet has been shown in studies to be effective in treating mood disorders such as bipolar disorder[64] and schizophrenia. In a case reported by Kraft and Westman at Duke University, a seventy-year-old woman with schizophrenia and a history of attempted suicide and psychotic behavior was put on a ketogenic diet for health reasons. Medications had not helped with symptoms, but, after eight days on the diet, she reported that the auditory and visual hallucinations she had been having since she was a child had gone away. She continued the diet, and, twelve months later, the hallucinations had not returned.[65]

- *Reduction of Factors Associated with Cancer:* As we have discussed, cancer cells depend on glucose to fuel themselves, and elevated levels of blood sugar and insulin increase the risks for developing cancer.[66] Researchers analyzed the data from the third National Health and Nutrition Examination Survey (NHANES) and found that "for every increase in 50 mg/dl of plasma glucose, there was a 22% increased risk of overall cancer mortality. Insulin resistance was associated with a 41% ... increased risk of overall cancer mortality."[67] A ketogenic diet reduces blood sugar and insulin dramatically and has been shown to have beneficial effects as a cancer therapy as ketogenic diets slow the growth of tumors by cutting off their fuel supply.[68]

- *Reduction of Inappropriate Hunger and Sugar Cravings:* Hunger is much easier to manage on a ketogenic diet as higher levels of blood ketones exert an appetite suppressing effect, partly through increased fuel flow to cells and partly because fat and protein are more substantial foods and take longer to digest.

A meta-analysis by Gibson et al. reported that individuals on a ketogenic diet reported less hunger and a reduced desire to eat.[69]

- *Weight Loss:* Ketogenic diets are effective for weight loss because they reduce hunger, blood-insulin levels and fat stores while increasing lean body mass. Insulin is a fat-storage hormone, and less insulin resistance means fat loss. One study by a team at Duke University showed that subjects following a ketogenic diet for six months lost an average of more than 10% of their body weight while improving cardiac risk factors without any adverse effects.[70] A study by a team at the University of Cincinnati reported that women in the low-carb diet arm of the study not only gained muscle mass but lost twice as much weight as fat mass than those in a low-fat diet group.[71]

- *Neurological Support and Protection:* Ketogenic diets exert a protective effect on brain function and brain cell (neuron) health through various mechanisms, including a reduction in inflammation, oxidative stress, and potent anti-seizure effects on nerve-cell chemicals called neurotransmitters. Studies have reported that the symptoms of neurological diseases such as dementia, Alzheimer's disease, Parkinson's disease, MS, epilepsy, and ALS can be improved using a ketogenic diet.[72,73]

As you can see from the list above, the temporary unpleasant effects of switching to a ketogenic diet are balanced nicely by the benefits that it bestows.

Monitoring Progress

Monitoring progress on a ketogenic diet involves three basic activities:

1. Having baseline laboratory blood tests performed periodically.
2. Monitoring your blood-glucose and ketone levels to determine how your food and supplement choices affect them.
3. Making adjustments and troubleshooting.

Keeping a food and supplement log and recording blood-glucose and ketone readings on a consistent basis are absolute musts. There is just no other way to understand the effect of your choices on blood glucose and ketone values without tracking what and how much you eat and what supplements you take. The other benefit of logging food, supplements, and blood measurements is having this information available to share with a health-care professional when you have trouble moving toward a G/K index of 1.0 or below.

Laboratory Tests

Most, if not all health practitioners will want to see the results of your laboratory tests as they work with you on the diet. In addition to your cancer-specific tumor-marker tests, the results of a liver-enzyme panel are helpful in determining liver-function issues that might interfere with the production of ketone bodies or impair your liver's ability to metabolize the high-fat intake associated with a ketogenic diet.

In addition, a complete blood count and full blood chemistry panel a helpful for checking for kidney and anemia issues. A lipid panel is used to check cholesterol and triglyceride levels, and you may also want to have your iron levels, magnesium levels, and vitamin D levels checked. Some practitioners also like to see a test done for vitamin B_{12} levels, especially if fatigue is a problem. Tests for inflammation may also be requested. This may include a C-Reactive Protein (CRP) test and other marker tests for oxidative stress, a potent driver of inflammation.

Finally, a hemoglobin A1c test (HbA1c) will provide a measure of average blood sugars over the previous three months. However, Miriam Kalamian warns that there are a number of health conditions common in people with cancer that can skew these test results. These include surgery, high red-blood-cell turnover, anemia, and a recent history of vitamin C infusions. Again, it is highly recommended that you find a qualified health-care practitioner to monitor your progress. Lab Tests Online is a good resource for understanding blood tests.

Measuring Blood-Glucose and Ketone Levels

Monitoring can be done with a glucose and ketone meter such as the Precision Xtra by Abbott Laboratories. If you have a choice, the Precision Xtra has been shown in studies to take more accurate readings. The meters are inexpensive, but ketone strips, in particular, are quite expensive. You can purchase the Precision Xtra ketone strips online from North Drug Mart for a more reasonable price. For the visually impaired, there's a meter called the Prodigy Voice, which gives results by sound.

Blood-glucose readings should be taken before breakfast, two hours after lunch, and a final daily reading two hours after the evening meal. Ketones should be tracked frequently at the start of the diet to ensure you are moving in the right direction. There are two recommended ways to test for ketones: urine tests or home blood meters. For the first two weeks of the diet, ketones can be tested using Bayer Ketostix, which measure urine levels of acetoacetate (AcAc). However, over time, this method is not as accurate as blood testing. After several weeks on the diet, the kidneys get better at reabsorbing AcAc, and the body begins converting most of the AcAc to beta-hydroxybutyrate (another type of ketone) that can be measured in the blood. Since Ketostixs test for acetoacetate, they won't be able to detect urine ketones accurately once the kidneys get better at reabsorbing acetoacetate. While these strips can be used for the first two weeks of the diet, afterward, a blood-ketone meter or laboratory test should be used.

If you are new to using a meter, I've established a webpage on ketogenic-diet-resource.com to provide help on checking your blood sugar with a meter[74]. Note that blood ketones tend to be lower in the morning and higher in the evening, while blood glucose is the opposite.

If you have trouble with glucose or ketone readings, check the troubleshooting section that follows for possible causes. Keep careful track of food, drinks, and supplements. Monitor your blood glucose both one hour and two hours after meals to see if what (or how much) you are eating is an issue, and tweak your diet and supplements accordingly. You can log this information on an Excel spreadsheet or in a hard-copy log or journal. The Wisconsin Diabetes Prevention website offers a useful log book you can download and print, or you can search for "blood sugar log" in Google or Bing and choose the one you like.

Troubleshooting Stubborn Blood-Glucose Levels

Lowering blood glucose and increasing ketone levels can be difficult even when following a strict ketogenic diet. Here are some points to consider if you are having trouble getting baseline blood-glucose levels to drop. My thanks to Miriam Kalamian for her assistance and expertise in these troubleshooting points.

- *Physical stress:* Cancer is a metabolic source of stress. Tumors may create metabolic waste products that can be converted to glucose. In addition, extensive liver metastases can interfere with the liver's ability to generate ketones.

- *Mental stress:* Excess emotional stress can increase levels of cortisol, a hormone that can increase blood glucose. Find ways to decrease emotional and mental stress: try yoga, prayer, meditation, art projects, or doing something that you love that absorbs your attention and takes your mind off of your health.

- *Chemotherapy and radiation:* Your body reacts to these treatments, just as it would react to any injury or illness, and blood glucose is increased. However, be aware that a ketogenic diet blunts this effect, so your blood sugar will be lower than it would be if you were eating a standard high-carb diet.

- *Medications:* Steroids and other drugs can increase blood sugar, but may be necessary for your treatment protocol. Talk to your primary care physician about equally effective drugs without this side effect.

- *Protein consumption:* It is very easy to "overeat" protein if food intake is not tracked via a food scale and log. At each meal, most people only need a serving of meat about two thirds the size of a deck of playing cards. Try lowering daily protein intake by ten grams (in other words, eat about 1.25 ounces less protein each day).

- *Hidden carbs:* Read labels and count every carb in food, drinks, and supplements. Sugar alcohols and excess fiber can cause blood-sugar spikes and interfere with ketosis for some people.

- *Carbohydrate intake on food labels:* Food labels do not provide accurate measures of carbohydrate. Food manufacturers can list zero carbs for up to 0.5 grams of carbohydrate per serving.

- *Vitamins, herbal supplements, toothpaste, lip balm and other cosmetic products:* These can have added sugars. Again, check labels. You may have to eliminate your supplements for several days while monitoring blood sugar. Then reintroduce them one at a time to determine which ones might be a source of hidden sugars.

- *Caffeine intake:* Drinking caffeinated coffee or sugar-free cocoa or eating dark chocolate and other caffeine-containing foods can drive up blood sugar.

- *Caloric intake:* Use the Customizing Your Diet steps in chapter 7 to find the recommended caloric intake for your ideal weight and adjust your caloric intake to match. If you are losing weight you don't want to lose, eat more calories, as too low of a caloric intake can also be a stressor that results in elevated blood sugar.

- *Exercise:* Moderate exercise can elevate blood sugar for a short time right after the exercise is stopped. However, it reduces baseline blood-glucose and insulin levels in the long run. In contrast, vigorous exercise can raise blood glucose for longer periods due to a stress response.

- *Intravenous vitamin C:* Intravenous C is metabolized like a carbohydrate, and in some situations, the administration of it can result in higher blood sugar.

- *Low thyroid function:* Check with your doctor on your thyroid status. Dr. Datis Kharrazian has an excellent book on this subject. Miriam Kalamian recommends that people with low thyroid function should ease into the ketogenic diet, one meal at a time. She suggests adding a quarter cup of cooked legumes or increasing the amounts of non-starchy vegetables at two meals until you adjust to a ketogenic diet plan.

- *Micronutrients:* Deficiencies of micronutrients can be detrimental to blood-sugar control. Taking at least a baseline multivitamin/multi-mineral is recommended. Vitamin D levels should also be checked and optimized. See supplement recommendations in appendix A.

- *Systemic body inflammation:* Inflammation can cause blood sugar to rise, so take steps to reduce it. Eat salmon, tuna or other oily fish more often or take fish or krill oil to increase omega-3 fatty acid intake. Herbs such as turmeric, ginger, garlic, cloves, cardamom and others are anti-inflammatory. Google "anti-inflammatory herbs" for more information.

- *Colds, flu and other illnesses:* Fighting off virus or bacterial infections will result in elevated blood sugars.

- *Insulin resistance:* As we age, most of us who are eating a standard high-carb diet can develop some sort of insulin resistance, a systemic body reaction to chronically high glucose and insulin levels. It takes time for this condition to reverse itself once a ketogenic diet is started.

- *Age in general:* Younger people will generally respond better to dietary changes with faster drops in blood glucose and higher ketones, often within days of starting the diet. Older people will find this process takes longer.

- *Gender:* Women can experience higher blood sugars during menstruation.

- *Blood measurement variations:* Home monitor readings may be higher than a venous blood draw at your doctor's office. Miriam writes, "ALL home monitors are merely screening tools developed for people with diabetes. That's why these 'generous' variations are considered acceptable. I took our meter to several of Raffi's blood draws and found that his venous draw analyzed at the lab was ALWAYS lower than the meter, so I factored that in when testing at home. Also, I advise people to take a second reading anytime the measurement looks either too high or too low." It also depends on the meter accuracy and various other factors so this is not written in stone.

Tips to Help You Start and Succeed

The tips below were developed over time and come from my own and other's individual experiences in implementing a ketogenic diet. They should help you achieve success as well.

- You must keep track of what you eat on a per-meal basis. Since the carbohydrate allowances are so small at the beginning of the diet, it's easy to eat too many. Protein must be tracked as well so as not to go over the daily recommended amount. Remember, excess protein can be converted into blood glucose, so stay within your limit. Keep a spreadsheet, use one of the web-based food-intake trackers, or keep a written log. I've provided one for you in appendix H. Not only will journaling help you accurately record food intake, it can also be used to track mood and physical changes for analysis should there be a need to troubleshoot. A journal is a good place to track blood-glucose and ketone levels as well.

- Recommended tools include Fitday.com, which offers both a web-based application and an application that can be downloaded to a PC. MyFitnessPal.com offers both a web-based and a mobile application. Cronometer.com is another good choice, so is FatSecret.com. The USDA's free nutrition database can also be utilized.[75] The Atkins.com website also has some nice tools for tracking progress on a ketogenic diet plan.

- Get a carb-counting guidebook or software application to learn how to count carbs in various foods. Counting net carbs is a crucial part of the diet, and it's important to understand how to do this correctly. *The Calorie King* book gets good reviews on Amazon, and it comes in both a paperback and a digital edition. *The Complete Book of Food Counts*, by Corrine Netzer is another good choice, as is Dana Carpender's *Carb and Calorie Counter*.

- Purchase a good quality digital food scale (accurate to at least 0.5 grams) so foods can be weighed and measured. This ensures accurate tracking of food amounts and calories.

- Go on a carbohydrate sweep. Inspect kitchen cupboards and refrigerator, removing or separating all high-carb foods. Restock or rearrange the kitchen so that low-carb, ketogenic foods are readily available. A low-carb food list is included in chapter 6 under the Allowed Foods section.

- Recognize that a ketogenic diet plan is not a "special diet" that requires special foods. Ketogenic foods are essentially real, whole foods close to their natural state. Avoid low-carb "convenience foods" such as shakes and bars. They are typically loaded with poor-quality proteins and sugar alcohols that can affect blood-glucose levels.

- Think about meal logistics, and learn to plan accordingly. This will help provide a framework to follow, starting with buying the right food at the grocery store. If proper foods have already been decided on for dinner, it will be easier to avoid making selections based on old habits.

- Replace old habits with new ones. If the normal routine is to visit the nearest coffee shop for a bagel, start making coffee at home and have it with eggs instead.

- Don't let travel situations put you in a bind. With low-carbohydrate diets increasing in popularity, you can find suitable options almost anywhere in a pinch. Most gas station convenience stores now carry nuts and sometimes even hard-boiled eggs. (See the Travel Tips section in chapter 9 for more information.)

- Avoid high-carb foods. I've included a list of these in the Foods to Avoid section in chapter 6. These are foods that drive up blood-glucose and insulin levels.

- Think about social situations that will be encountered, and devise ways to handle temptations to eat the "old" way. This will help with the problem of being blindsided when someone at the office brings in a box of cookies. Likewise, a beer with friends usually turns into a date with potato skins and nachos. Think salad and steak instead.

- Be prepared to spend more time in the kitchen. This is an important point. A ketogenic diet involves cooking and eating real foods. Those who are not accustomed to preparing meals will find that this is a good time to learn about cooking in general and specifically ketogenic cooking.

- Stay hydrated. As carb intake is lowered, your kidneys will start dumping excess water. In addition, you need plenty of water to work toward lower blood-sugar readings. At the very least, make sure to drink enough water to replace what is lost. A good general rule is to drink half the number of pounds of your ideal body weight in ounces of water each day. If your ideal weight is 150 pounds, try to drink seventy-five ounces of water each day. Broths without MSG (monosodium glutamate) are good choices for hydration because they also provide minerals.

- Don't be afraid to eat more fat. Many people have trouble on a ketogenic diet plan because they just can't get past the idea that eating lots of fat, especially saturated animal fat is bad. To complicate the issue, particularly if total cholesterol goes up while on the diet, uninformed physicians may voice concerns about this. The underlying fear has to do with the messages in the media (and from the mainstream medical industry), who are still holding onto the myth that saturated fat and cholesterol are the cause of heart disease. This is old thinking, and there is now a large volume of research that indicates that saturated fat and cholesterol have no correlation to heart disease or any other health issue. In reality, the more damaging factors in body health are elevated insulin and blood sugar.

- Talk with household members and let them know there are certain foods that are required for adherence to the diet. It makes the diet more difficult to follow if you find the dinner you had prepared has been eaten by someone else in the house.

- Manage protein intake. This is perhaps the most difficult task on a ketogenic diet. A normal breakfast of two eggs and four sausage links adds up to twenty-eight grams of protein, a relatively large intake for one meal. In addition, standard cancer treatments may cause side effects that make it difficult to eat protein foods. In these cases, protein powders may be recommended by a health-care professional. Miriam Kalamian sometimes uses protein powders as a meal replacement for individuals having difficulty with consuming and digesting whole-protein foods. She emphasizes the need to stay within the protein limits set for the individual. A fat or oil should also be added to slow absorption and to keep the ratio of fats to carbs and proteins in the proper ketogenic range.

6

• • •

Food Facts, Fasting and What to Eat

Nutrient intake on a ketogenic diet targeted for cancer treatment typically adheres to the following guidelines:

- 78%–86% calories from fats

- 9%–11% calories from proteins

- 2%–4% calories from carbohydrates

These ratios, along with intermittent fasting (if needed), should help you achieve a desirable G/K index. As one might imagine, the recommended ratios are not written in stone. In particular, percentages of macronutrients will vary as calorie intake varies. In addition, individual responses differ, and adjustments will need to be made based on test results from blood glucose and ketone monitoring.

About Fats

Let's talk about fats as they constitute the majority of calories on the diet. There are several types of fats and oils, which have different effects on the body. These fall into three major groups, depending on their chemical structure: saturated fats, monounsaturated fats, and polyunsaturated fats.

Saturated fats are those which are solid at room temperature, such as butter and coconut oil. These fats are the most stable chemically and the least inflammatory.

Monounsaturated fats are liquid at room temperature and somewhat stable chemically. These include olive oil and other types of fats such as oleic acid, which is found in mayonnaise, beef tallow, and olive oil.

Polyunsaturated fats such as omega-6 and omega-3 fatty acids are the least stable of all of the fat types. The omega-6 fats such as vegetable oils, legumes and nuts tend to have an inflammatory result in the body. The famous omega-3 fats (found in fish oil and in fatty fish) are also polyunsaturated and less stable, but they have an anti-inflammatory effect on the body through the activation of different metabolic pathways. Small amounts of omega-3 fats can be used to reduce inflammation.

Since the majority of calories on a ketogenic diet will come from dietary fats, they should be chosen with digestive tolerance in mind. Saturated and monounsaturated fats such as butter, macadamia nuts, coconut oil, olive oil, avocado and egg yolks are tolerated more easily by most people. In addition, these fats are more chemically stable, so they don't contribute to inflammation. Most people cannot tolerate eating large amounts of polyunsaturated vegetable oils. Examples of foods high in omega-6 fatty acids include mayonnaise, margarine, soybean oil, sunflower oil, safflower oil, corn oil and canola oil. Most nuts (with the exception of macadamias) are high in omega-6 fatty acids, so go easy on them.

Your intake of polyunsaturated fats should also be balanced between omega-6 and omega-3 types. Omega-3 fats can be found in fatty fish such as anchovies, sardines, salmon and tuna, walnuts, flaxseeds, and grass-fed meats. In other words, emphasize fish and grass-fed meat and limit vegetable oils and nuts in your meals.

Fats and oils can be added to meals in the form of sauces such as hollandaise, full-fat salad dressings, and dips made from sour cream. Over time, it will become a habit to add a source of fat to each meal.

Coconut Oil

Coconut oil is a particularly important source of fat on a ketogenic diet. In addition to being a source of long-chain fatty acids, it also contains natural medium-chain triglycerides (MCTs). MCTs have a chemical structure that allows them to bypass normal fatty-acid digestion pathways. Instead, MCTs are passed directly from the intestinal tract to the liver and are broken down immediately into ketone bodies. The addition of small amounts of coconut oil to your diet will help elevate ketones quickly. However, relying on coconut oil for all of your fat intake is not recommended. Be sure to include butter, ghee, olive oil and animal fats in your daily intake.

Organic, cold pressed extra-virgin coconut oil is much more available now than it used to be. There are many different brands, and you can buy it online at several online stores. Just google organic coconut oil. I have the Nutiva brand and feel it has a better flavor than Tropical Traditions' product. Another one of my favorites is Artisana's coconut butter. A spoonful right out of the jar is just so good.

MCT Oil

MCT oil is a special supplemental oil composed entirely of medium-chain triglycerides. It can be taken at the start of the diet to provide a ketone source while your body makes the adjustments necessary to create ketones internally. Start slowly with small amounts of MCT and coconut oil, as too much can cause gastric distress, and don't use MCT oil as your only fat source. Some people have reported that too much MCT causes stress reactions such as heart palpitations.

Dairy Fats and Dairy Proteins

One of the questions I am asked about this diet most often is why dairy protein is restricted, but dairy fat is acceptable. Here's why.

Dairy products high in protein (cheese, milk, yogurt) contain a specific type of protein called casein. They also contain lactose, which is a form of milk sugar. Both of these constituents have insulin-stimulating properties, meaning that when we eat them, they cause insulin to increase in the bloodstream. This is the opposite of what we want for cancer patients, so some ketogenic experts advise that dairy proteins be avoided to minimize insulin spikes.

However, dairy fats (butter, sour cream, heavy cream, and cream cheese) have minimal amounts of casein and lactose since they are mostly fat. Therefore, they have less effect on insulin levels. Since it's challenging to successfully follow a ketogenic diet without dairy fats, I advise they be eaten in small amounts. Dr. Dominic D'Agostino recommends limiting dairy fats to a range of twenty to thirty percent of total calories. You can test your response to eating them and adjust the amounts accordingly to maintain optimal blood-sugar and ketone levels.

One caveat on dairy consumption comes from my colleague Patricia Daly in Ireland. She reports that chemotherapy treatments can cause a temporary lactose and fructose (fruit sugar) intolerance, so cancer patients receiving chemotherapy may need to avoid dairy until after treatments have stopped and a gut-healing regimen has been successful.

In addition, many people have concerns about the amount of hormones in dairy products, having read on the Internet that they can contribute to cancer. In studying published research papers that report steroid hormones in animal products, it's clear that the amount of hormones in the food we eat is miniscule in comparison to the amount of steroid hormones our own bodies make on a daily basis. In addition, the digestive process likely breaks down the hormones before they ever reach our bloodstream.[75]

I also looked at research on the effects of dairy product consumption on cancers. The latest review of the evidence by a team from the University of Copenhagen in

Denmark was published in November 2016, and it found no association between dairy consumption and cancer. The authors stated that

> *"Among cancers, milk and dairy intake was inversely associated with colorectal cancer, bladder cancer, gastric cancer, and breast cancer, and not associated with risk of pancreatic cancer, ovarian cancer, or lung cancer, while the evidence for prostate cancer risk was inconsistent."*[77]

This is not to say there is no link, because we don't have enough data to make that conclusion. There are epidemiological studies that link milk consumption to various cancers, but these studies are large cohorts in which the study authors try to find an association by looking at rates of disease in general populations that eat dairy. Only specific controlled clinical trials can provide definitive data, and there is no data from any specific controlled clinical trial that supports these general epidemiological associations.

Hence, at this point I don't think the research is strong enough either way to make a determination. If you are suspicious about dairy, don't include it in your diet. There are many websites that offer dairy-free low-carb recipes if you enter that search term into Google. I include dairy fats in this book because I think it's tough to get fat intake high enough without them, and I haven't seen any definitive clinically relevant evidence to support a dairy-consumption link to cancer.

Protein and Amino Acids

Proteins in the body are created from the amino acid building blocks that come from the digestion of protein-containing foods. The body can make many of twenty basic amino acids it requires for good health, however, eight amino acids are essential, meaning the body cannot make them so they must be obtained from the foods we eat. Getting enough protein is important because protein plays a role in just about every metabolic process in the human body, and it's required for retaining lean muscle tissue when carbohydrate intake is restricted.

While on a ketogenic diet, protein intake (meat, fish, poultry, and eggs) is controlled but adequate, meaning just enough is allowed on a daily basis to support and maintain muscle mass. If you reduce your carbohydrate intake but continue to eat more protein than you need for maintaining body tissues, the excess amino acids can result in higher blood-glucose levels. In addition, cancer cells can use the excess amounts of certain amino acids, such as glutamine, as a substitute fuel source.

Keep in mind that we cannot eliminate protein from our diet completely. We must eat some each day because protein is an essential nutrient, and we must have it in our diet to sustain life. The strategy of the diet is to provide just enough protein to maintain health but not too much. It's really a matter of balance, not avoidance.

About Glutamine

Glutamine is an amino acid found in all animal foods and dairy proteins. It is required for good health. However, it also happens to be an amino acid that human cells, including cancer cells, can use as an energy source, and it is also the reason that a ketogenic diet doesn't stop cancer completely. Cancer cells are stubbornly resourceful, and using glutamine is one way they can continue to thrive even when carbohydrate-based fuels are restricted. It would seem that avoiding glutamine would be a good strategy in treating cancer with a ketogenic diet. However, the truth is that it's very difficult to remove glutamine from your diet entirely, as you require foods, such as meat, poultry and fish, which contain it. In fact, if you try to avoid glutamine in your diet, your body will use other amino acids to make the glutamine it needs, so again, it's really a strategy of balance, not avoidance.

Limiting total protein intake helps with that balance. By restricting total protein intake to the amount needed to support body maintenance, you get enough glutamine but not too much. The customized planning steps you'll follow in chapter 7 to determine your macronutrients will help you determine the correct amount of protein to eat for your individual needs.

L-Glutamine Supplement Recommendations

L-glutamine supplements and whey protein powders containing large amounts of glutamine are generally not recommended, although much of the glutamine in these products is absorbed by cells lining the intestinal wall and in the liver. For this reason, some practitioners recommend glutamine supplementation to help heal the gut if it has been damaged by traditional chemotherapy and radiation treatments, reasoning that most of it will be absorbed in the gut, and not spill over into the blood stream. However, the research on this is not definitive. Dr. D'Agostino's team has the investigation of this topic on their research agenda for the near future.

For now, in this publication, avoiding glutamine supplementation is recommended. In addition, it's also a good idea to read labels and also avoid MSG, hydrolyzed vegetable protein, soy protein, and aspartame as these are sources of glutamate, which is derived from glutamine

Carbohydrates

Carbohydrates are sugars and starches. Sugars, starches, and sugar alcohols are hidden in all kinds of processed foods and are listed with many alternate names. Be diligent about reading labels to find hidden carbohydrate sources. You may recognize some of these common names:

- Sugars are glucose, fructose, sucrose, honey, dextrose, molasses, corn sugar, corn syrup, high-fructose corn syrup, fruit-juice concentrate, cane juice, treacle, lactose, galactose, maltose, maltodextrin, hydrolyzed starch, demerara, turbinado, maple syrup, agave syrup.

- Starches are corn starch, vegetable starch, arrowroot, cassava, amaranth, barley, wheat, wheat starch, buckwheat, corn, HVP, HPP, malt, millet, modified food starch, oats, potato, quinoa, rice, sorghum, spelt, teff, tapioca, triticale.

- Sugar alcohols are polydextrose, glycerin, maltitol, mannitol, sorbitol, xylitol, erythritol, glycerol, isomalt, lactitol, inositol.

Generally, any chemical name with an ose ending is a sugar, and any chemical name ending with an ol is a sugar alcohol.

Although they do contain small amounts of healthy nutrients, most fruits and many vegetables are also high in carbohydrate. Green leafy vegetables are the lowest in carbohydrate, but they do still have enough carbohydrate to count. Since carb allowances and target levels of blood glucose are so very low at the start of the diet, you must be diligent about counting carbs in every food that you eat or drink. Even the use of daily cosmetic and hygiene products should be as carb-free as possible.

As best you can, take into account any carbohydrates in supplements, medicines, chewing gums, toothpaste and even skin products. As an illustration of how important this is, I have read about epilepsy patients having seizures because they put lotion containing sorbitol on their skin. The absorption of sorbitol, a sugar alcohol, interferes with ketosis. For this reason, the Charlie Foundation, an organization that supports and encourages the use of ketogenic diets as a treatment, has a list of commercial products that are safe for use by people with epilepsy. This list should also be helpful to those who are using a ketogenic diet as a cancer therapy.[78]

Don't rely on food labels. Food manufacturers naturally have an interest in underreporting the number of carbs in their products. Remember to check serving sizes as well. When looking at a container of yogurt that has 16 carbohydrates per serving, verify the number of servings in the container. If there are two servings, then the total carb count for that container is 32 carbs, not 16.

Calculating Total versus Net Carbs

An important point to understand about carb restriction is the difference between the measure of total carbohydrate and the measure of "net" carbs. The difference is the amount of fiber in the food. Fiber is an indigestible form of carbohydrate, and it has a minimal effect on blood glucose since humans cannot digest and absorb it. To measure carbohydrates correctly, subtract fiber from the total carbohydrate count. Total carb is the count of all carbohydrate grams available in the food, including fiber, sugar alcohols, and other indigestible carbohydrates.

Net carbs is the total carb count in grams minus grams of indigestible fiber. Most carb-counting books will include a measurement of total-carb grams, fiber grams and then the net carb grams. (Net carbs can also be referred to as "effective" or "usable" carbs.)

To count carbs accurately, use the net-carbs numbers when adding up carbohydrate intake. All foods should be weighed and measured to obtain accurate carb counts. There are many sources of information that give carb and net-carb counts for various foods. (See the Tips to Help You Start and Succeed section in chapter 5 for recommendations.)

Increasing Carb Limits over Time

Once your blood sugars and ketones are close to or below a G/K index of 1.0, you can slowly begin to add carbohydrates back into your diet in 5 gram increments, holding at each new level for one week. However, you must keep track of blood sugar and ketones while adding carbohydrate to your diet so that you can determine your "carb-tolerance limit." If baseline blood sugar goes up or ketones drop after a carb addition, you have surpassed your carb tolerance. Return to your previous carb limit and remain there.

To clarify with an example, after you reach a G/K index of 1.0, you could then raise daily carbs to a 17-gram limit for one week. If glucose and ketone test levels are not affected, then at the start of the second week, you could raise your daily limit to 22 carb grams per day. Repeat this process until you hit your carb tolerance. Also, if you want to keep your calorie intake the same as you increase carbohydrate, simply reduce your daily fat intake by a tablespoon or two. Do not lower protein intake to save calories.

Fiber

Ketogenic diets can be low in fiber. If you feel you need fiber, focus on sources of both soluble and insoluble fiber. Increase fiber intake by adding chia seeds or ground flaxseed to meals. Romaine lettuce can be used to add bulk fiber to the diet, as can spinach or kale.

If you prefer to take fiber separately, try a gentle soluble fiber such as psyllium husk. Plain psyllium husk is recommended, as products such as Metamucil or its generic equivalents have carb-containing fillers. Also, psyllium may reduce or delay the absorption of certain medications. As a rule, don't take psyllium supplements at the same time as you take other medication or supplements. Take psyllium at least one hour before or two to four hours after taking other medications.

Be aware that psyllium husk is not recommended for people with ulcerative colitis or adhesions, or if you have difficulty swallowing. Also, never start psyllium if you are constipated, as it can cause an intestinal obstruction. In any event, it's best to introduce it slowly:

- Begin with 1/2 teaspoon in eight ounces of warm water once a day. Mix well, and then it drink immediately before it becomes too thick to swallow comfortably. (Psyllium thickens rapidly when added to water.)

- Over time, increase to the amount that works for you. Most experts recommend two teaspoons in two large glasses of water per day, as needed.

- Always take psyllium with a full glass of water, and drink at least six to eight glasses of water throughout the day to avoid constipation.

Water and Dehydration

Everyone needs water to replace what the body loses through daily activity. On a ketogenic diet, it is even more important, since the diet has a diuretic effect.

Drinking plenty of water also helps to remove metabolic waste from the body and supports many different metabolic functions. It's logical that water is lost when you urinate or sweat, but you may not realize that small amounts of water are lost each time you exhale. You need to replace this lost water to prevent dehydration. I can't emphasize enough how important it is that you drink plenty of water.

In addition, your body will need more water if you live in a hot or dry climate, are more physically active, are sick and running a fever, or have diarrhea or are vomiting. Some people may have fluid restrictions because of health problems such as heart or kidney disease. If your health care provider has told you to restrict fluid intake, be sure to follow that advice.

Allowed Foods

The short story on allowed foods is to get the recommended amount of protein each day, limit carbohydrates, and fill in the rest of your calories with fats and oils. The lists below should help you choose appropriate foods in each macronutrient category.

Sources of Protein

Fattier cuts of meat are better because they contain less protein and more fat. Choose wild-caught seafood, organic eggs, and organic or grass-fed animal foods when possible to minimize bacteria, antibiotic, and steroid-hormone intake. Websites such as www. eatwild.com or www.localharvest.org can help with locating local sources of clean, grass-fed meats and poultry. Consider this wide range of protein sources:

- *Whole eggs:* these can be prepared in various ways. Try deviled, fried, hard-boiled, omelets, poached, scrambled, and soft-boiled.

- *Meat:* all cuts of beef, pork, lamb, veal, and goat. Look out for added sugar in hams and prepared deli meats. Fattier cuts of meat are better because they contain less protein and more fat.

- *Game meat:* venison, elk, buffalo/bison, and other wild game are good sources of protein, although these meats are usually lower in fat than beef and pork.

- *Organ meats/offal:* organ meats such as liver and heart are extremely nutritious. Roasted marrow bones are an especially fat-rich culinary treat.

- *Poultry:* chicken, turkey, quail, Cornish hen, duck, goose, and pheasant. Free range is better, if it's available. Dark meat is better because of the higher fat content. There is no need to purchase skinless poultry. The skin is rich in fat and protein, and when roasted until crispy, it's delicious! You will also find that skin-on, bone-in poultry is more economical than boneless, skinless cuts.

- *Fish of any kind:* anchovies, calamari, catfish, cod, flounder, halibut, herring, mackerel, mahi-mahi, salmon, sardines, scrod, sole, snapper, trout, and tuna. When buying canned salmon and sardines, favor varieties with the bones and skin. The bones provide minerals, and the skin provides more of the important omega-3 fats. (Exceptions include breaded and fried seafood, which are high in carbohydrates.)

- *Shellfish and seafood:* clams, crab, lobster, scallops, shrimp, squid, mussels, and oysters. (The exception is imitation crab meat; it often contains sugar and gluten.)

- *Bacon and sausage:* check labels and avoid those cured with excessive sugar (maple flavor for example) or containing fillers such as textured vegetable protein (TVP), soy isolate, wheat gluten, or milk protein. Specialty health-food stores carry most brands of sugar-free and filler-free bacon and sausage. Each serving should have no more than one carb.

- *Protein powders:* rice, pea, hemp, or other vegetable protein powders can be used occasionally, but read the labels for added sugars. Also, don't rely on them exclusively as a protein source, and unless recommended by your healthcare professional, avoid whey, as it elevates insulin. The TrueNutrition.com website has been recommended for vegetarian protein powders.

- *Nuts and seeds:* macadamias are the highest in fat and lowest in carbohydrate. Pecans, almonds, and walnuts are good choices. Cashews are higher in carbs so track intake carefully to avoid going over your carbohydrate limits.

Here's a note about fried pork rinds: they have zero carbohydrate and can be used as an occasional snack; however, the protein in them does not contain all of the necessary amino acids. Count the protein grams but limit the amount so as not to displace other complete-protein foods.

Fats and Oils

As discussed in the About Fats section earlier, saturated and monounsaturated fats are healthier overall. I've marked each item below as to whether they are mostly saturated (S), monounsaturated (M), or polyunsaturated (P). In addition, avoid hydrogenated fats, such as margarine, to minimize trans-fat intake. If you use vegetable oils (olive, canola, sunflower, safflower, soybean, flaxseed and sesame oils) select "cold-pressed" organic brands. Keep cold-pressed oils, like almond and flaxseed, refrigerated to minimize rancidity. Avoid heating vegetable oils. Use clean, non-hydrogenated lard, beef tallow, coconut oil, and ghee for frying, since they have higher smoke points.

- Avocado. (M)
- Avocado oil. (M)
- Almond oil. (P,M)
- Beef tallow (can be obtained online), preferably from grass fed cattle. (S, M)
- Butter: try to find organic sources. (S)
- Organic chicken or duck fat can be obtained online. (S,M)
- Ghee is butter with milk solids removed. (S)
- Lard that is not hydrogenated. (S,M)

- Macadamia nuts. (M)
- Macadamia oil. (M)
- Mayonnaise, no or low sugar. Duke's brand is sugar free. (P)
- Olive oil, organic. (M)
- Olives, green and black. (M)
- Organic coconut oil, coconut butter and coconut cream concentrate. (S)
- Organic red palm oil. (S)
- Peanut butter, make sure to use unsweetened products, and limit due to omega-6 content. (P,M)
- Seed and most nut oils. (P)
- Dark chocolate (90 percent cocoa) can be used in very small amounts. (S, M)

Fresh Vegetables

Most non-starchy vegetables are low in carbs and are good choices. Choose organic vegetables to avoid pesticide residues. Sweeter vegetables such as onions, shallots, tomatoes, carrots, peppers, and summer squashes are marked with an asterisk (*) as they are relatively high in carbohydrate, so track them closely. If you choose frozen or canned products, read labels to make sure no sugar is added. This list is not exhaustive, so if you have other favorites, and they fit your carb limits, please enjoy them.

- Alfalfa sprouts
- Any leafy green vegetable
- Asparagus
- Avocado
- Bamboo shoots
- Bean sprouts
- Beet greens
- Bell peppers*
- Bok choy
- Broccoli
- Brussels sprouts
- Cabbage
- Carrots*
- Cauliflower
- Celery
- Celery root
- Chives
- Collard greens
- Cucumbers
- Dandelion greens
- Fennel
- Garlic
- Kale
- Kohlrabi
- Leeks
- Lettuces and salad greens (arugula, chicory, fennel, mache, endive, escarole, Boston lettuce, radicchio, romaine, sorrel)
- Mushrooms
- Olives
- Onions*
- Radishes
- Sauerkraut
- Scallions
- Shallots*
- Snow peas
- Spinach
- Sprouts
- Summer squash*
- Swiss chard
- Tomatoes*
- Turnips

Dairy Fats

Try to obtain organic products from grass-fed animals, which are generally healthier.

- Full-fat sour cream. Check labels for additives and fillers. Look for brands, such as Daisy, that are pure cream with no added milk or whey.
- Butter. Kerrygold brand is recommended if you can find it.
- Cream cheese (Look for brands without added whey.)
- Marscapone cheese
- Ghee. (This is butter with the milk solids removed.)
- Heavy whipping cream. (at least 36 percent milk fat content).

Beverages

Beverages should be unsweetened and decaffeinated. Caffeine is restricted because it can increase blood glucose. Be sure to check labels to avoid added sweeteners. Include any protein grams in your daily protein total.

- Water.
- Clear broth or bouillon (no added MSG).
- Lemon or lime juice in small amounts.
- Decaf coffee.
- Decaf black tea.
- Herbal tea.
- Flavored seltzer water.
- Almond milk.
- Soy milk.
- Coconut milk, canned or refrigerated carton.

Sweeteners

Avoiding sweetened foods in general will help "reset" the taste buds. However, if there is a desire for something sweet, there are recommended choices for sweeteners. Note that the powdered forms of most artificial sweeteners usually have maltodextrin, dextrose, or some other sugar added, so liquid products are preferred.

- *Stevia: liquid stevia or stevia glycerite.* The SweetLeaf brand is good, but any of the liquid products should be fine. Stevia has a "licorice" back taste if you use too much, especially with the powdered form. Stevia is extremely concentrated, so a tiny pinch of the powder or just a few drops of the liquid go a long way. Use a light hand until you gauge the proper amount for your taste. Some users have found that if you mix artificial sweeteners, the taste is better, and you can use less to get the same sweet taste.

- *Splenda:* This is the brand name of sucralose and the EZ-Sweet brand is recommended. The smaller bottle is very concentrated; just one drop will sweeten a whole cup of tea. However, any liquid sucralose product will work. Even for the liquid sweeteners, read the labels and check to make sure no sugar such as cane syrup, dextrose or maltodextrin is blended into the product that you choose.

- *Special note on sugar alcohols such as xylitol and erythritol:* These sweeteners are low carb, and they don't affect blood glucose. However, in several older studies, sugar alcohols have demonstrated an "anti-ketogenic" effect, meaning they interfere with ketosis, so it's best to avoid them while on the diet. I have seen real evidence of this in my own ketone testing.

In my opinion, eating sugar, honey, and other nutritive sweeteners has a negative effect on blood sugar which surpasses those that might be associated with using a small amount of Splenda or any other non-nutritive sweetener. However, I also believe this is an individual decision. If any sweetener or other food product causes problems for you, avoid consuming it.

Spices

Spices do have carbs, so be sure to count them if they are added to meals in more than tiny amounts. Also, commercial spice mixes like steak seasoning or Greek seasoning usually have added sugar, as do flavored extracts. I've included a table at the end of appendix G that contains the carb counts of various dried spices and flavored extracts.

Foods to Avoid

In general, foods which are rich in carbohydrates, casein (milk protein), and lactose (milk sugar) are the foods to avoid.

Sugars and Sweetened Foods

Sugar is ever-present in our food supply and not only in candy, soft drinks, and fruit jams and spreads. The only way to truly avoid it is to only eat fresh, unprocessed foods such as meats, poultry, seafood, eggs, nuts and green leafy vegetables. If packaged foods are consumed, read the food labels carefully. Avoid any foods that have been sweetened. Watch out for these sugars:

- Sugars: white sugar (sucrose), brown sugar, cane sugar, powdered sugar.
- Evaporated cane juice or cane syrup.
- Crystalline fructose.
- Syrups: corn syrup, sorghum, honey, maple syrup, agave.
- Simple sugars: maltose, fructose, glucose, lactose.
- Sugar alcohols such as sorbitol, xylitol, erythritol, mannitol and maltitol. Natural sugar alcohol sweeteners have been shown in studies to be "anti-ketogenic" and can derail the process of ketosis, so avoid them if possible.
- Avoid the obvious sweet foods: cakes, cookies, muffins, pies, but also look out for foods like ketchup, soup, bread, and even canned vegetables. Sugar is added to most processed canned, frozen or dried foods.

Processed and Convenience Foods

These foods contain plenty of chemical preservatives, MSG, hidden sugars and other carbohydrates:

- Chips made from potatoes or other starchy vegetables. (This includes Terra chips, vegetable chips, crunchy bean pods, and the like.)
- Canned soups and stews. (Most canned products contain hidden starchy thickeners.)
- Bagged and boxed processed foods—Hamburger Helper, stuffing mixes, puddings, Jello gelatin, etc. (Most are high in wheat or sugar and contain added chemicals in the forms of preservatives and fillers.)

All Grains and Grain Products

Wheat flour is also widely used as a filler in processed foods. Read the food labels carefully, and avoid any foods that contain the following: wheat, barley, rye, sorghum, triticale, teff, spelt, rice, vegetable protein, amaranth, buckwheat, millet, quinoa, corn.

- Products made from grain flours: white flour, whole-wheat flour, bread flour, oat flour, teff flour, rice flour, soy flour, breads of all kinds, waffles, pancakes, pasta, muffins, cold cereals, hot cereals, bread crumbs, flour tortillas, crackers, cookies, cakes, pies, pretzels, wraps, flatbread, etc.
- Corn products, including: cornbread, tamales, corn chips, grits, polenta, popcorn, corn tortillas, stuffing mixes and cornmeal. Corn is in most processed foods as high-fructose corn syrup or as a thickener or a preservative.

Starchy Vegetables

- Potatoes and other starchy tubers—sweet potatoes and potato products, such as hash browns, potato chips, tater tots, and French fries.
- Corn, lima beans, peas, okra, and artichokes.

Dairy Proteins

Normally, clean, organic dairy protein foods are good sources of nutrition, but it is best to avoid them on the ketogenic diet for the following reasons:

- Milk contains lactose (milk sugar) and casein (a milk protein), and both increase insulin levels.
- Fermented milk products like cheese and yogurt are lower in lactose, but they are also rich in casein, so it is best to avoid or limit them.
- Milk-based whey protein powders should be avoided or limited unless they are specifically recommended by a health-care professional. Rice, pea, hemp or other vegetable protein powders are acceptable. The TrueNutrition.com website has been recommended for vegetarian protein powders.

Fruit and Fruit Products

While they do have some health benefits, fruits in any form (dried, fresh, frozen) are high in carbs and fructose. Fructose, even from natural fruit, places a metabolic load on the liver and can drive up blood glucose if eaten in large amounts.

- Bananas, grapes, oranges, peaches and dried fruit are the highest in carbohydrate. Avoid them as they will sharply increase blood glucose.
- Berries are the lowest in carbohydrate. If the craving for something sweet becomes overwhelming, you could try a few strawberries, blueberries or raspberries, and then test two hours later to see if they significantly lower ketone levels or increase blood glucose.

Beverages

- Non-diet sodas: sodas often contain large amounts of high-fructose corn syrup (HFCS), which stresses and impairs liver function. However, if you want a sweet tasting soda, try the Zevia brand, which is made with stevia, or the Hanson's diet brand, which uses Splenda. I personally love the fizz of flavored sparkling water and sometimes add liquid stevia for a "soda" experience.

- Sweet alcohol sources such as liquors, sweet drinks and dessert wines.
- Malt beverages and beers.
- Juices made from fruit and vegetables, which are very high in sugar. (Several tablespoons of lemon or lime juice are okay.)
- Milk should be avoided due to the high casein and lactose content. These substances increase blood glucose and insulin.
- Sweetened varieties of almond and coconut milk.

Reading Food Labels

Food labels can be misleading, and you'll find, over time, that it's easier to just avoid commercially processed foods. These foods almost always contain starch, sugar or MSG in some form. For example, taco seasoning packets often include wheat flour and sugar in the form of dextrose and maltodextrin. Spaghetti sauce or alfredo sauce in glass jars frequently contains food starch, sugar and dried whey, plus autolyzed yeast extract, another form of MSG.

In addition, be sure to look at the serving size and then total carbohydrate amounts on the labels. The serving size might be written as a ¼ cup, but most people would use a larger serving. Remember, to calculate net carbs, simply take the total carbs and subtract the fiber carbs.

Fasting and Intermittent Fasting

The decision to begin a ketogenic diet depends on the individual's health and on a willingness to take up the challenge of the diet. There are various methods discussed in medical literature on the best way to begin. Some health-care professionals recommend starting slowly, reducing carbohydrate intake to below 50 grams per day and then reducing it further after a few weeks. This may be the safest and most comfortable way for those with severe insulin resistance (IR), since it will minimize the discomfort of hypoglycemic reactions that may occur.

Dr. Seyfried has recommended that individuals who are relatively strong[79] can start the diet with a forty-eight- to seventy-two-hour fast to quickly lower blood glucose and raise ketone levels. However, if the individual is underweight or malnourished for any reason, fasting is not recommended, as further weight loss may compromise health. Underweight, for our purposes here, is defined as having a body mass index (BMI) below 22.[80]

Although fasting has positive effects (lower blood levels of insulin and IGF-1) it can also cause an increase in stress hormones, especially for women, and slow thyroid function, as the body will automatically slow metabolism to conserve energy. This is especially true if the individual is also exercising while fasting. For those who don't feel that multiple-day fasting is for them, Dr. Seyfried and Dr. Dominic D'Agostino at the University of South Florida have also recommended intermittent fasting to help increase ketone levels and reduce blood glucose by aiding in the depletion of glycogen stores.

Intermittent fasting (IF) can take the form of skipping a meal or two.[80] For example, having breakfast the first day, and not eating again until dinner time that day or waiting longer until breakfast the second day. However, be aware that over time there may be a difference in response to this type of fasting based on gender. Women may not benefit as much as men when utilizing fasting or IF. The human research data is scarce, but some studies show fasting increases metabolic stress for female animals. This may be related to reproductive factors. In other words, because females are the child-bearing gender, there may be stress-related hormonal changes that slow metabolism even further in an attempt to protect reproduction capabilities. However, this is another individual response issue. In other words, your mileage may vary.

Fasting Tips

If you are a strong and relatively healthy individual and you would like to implement a fast as a kick start to the ketogenic diet, here are some tips that may help:

- When hunger threatens, get busy doing something else to help wait it out. On the first day of the fast, hunger will be persistent, but I find that it subsides toward the end of that day, presumably because ketone levels increase.

- Keep your mind occupied during fasting days. Plan to do something that is really engaging and takes your full attention.

- Drink lots of water, and take the vitamin and mineral supplements recommended in appendix A each day of the fast. Stomach cramping can occur if you don't drink enough water, so be sure to stay hydrated.

- Along with the water, you will need salt and potassium. A lack of these minerals may manifest as a headache or lightheadedness. You can make homemade mineral water (see appendix A) and sip that throughout the day, or take one buffered electrolyte capsule, such as Succeed S! Caps, as symptoms arise.

- Start the fast by taking blood-glucose and ketone readings the first morning. Then take readings in the evening, and repeat this the next day. It's motivational to see the numbers start moving toward the target ranges.

- For many people, the morning readings of blood glucose will be higher, but ketones will be lower. This is due to gluconeogenesis during the night. I've found that this will cause a transient increase in hunger, which subsides as the day goes on.

- If you are a coffee drinker or have a sweet tooth, the fast will go much easier if you take a few days to wean yourself off these foods before starting. I can't emphasize this enough. The side effects of coming off these addictive substances will make you miserable even when you aren't fasting. You don't want to compound the difficulty.

- You may experience some hypoglycemic symptoms such as a dull headache, heart palpitations, shakiness, dizziness and a feeling of being light-headed. These are normal responses to an adrenalin-based warning from the brain that blood glucose is low. Drink some homemade mineral water, and try to wait it out. (See Side Effect 1 in chapter 4.)

- After the fast is over, eat small amounts and take it easy when reintroducing food. Your digestive tract will be happier.

I recommend you pick a three-day period where you will be quite busy but be at home where you can control your exposure to food. Being at work is distracting but there are many pitfalls, especially in the break room where someone always has a box of cookies or doughnuts available.

My Personal Experience with Fasting

In writing this book, I thought it only fair that I should practice the ideas that I recommend, so I put myself on a three-day fast and then followed the dietary recommendations for several days afterward. These are my results:

- Hunger was manageable. I follow a low-carbohydrate diet most of the time, so I'm already somewhat adapted to ketosis. If you have never eaten a low-carbohydrate diet, reducing your sugar, flour and caffeine intake for four to five days before you start will make that first fasting day much easier.

- I had dinner at 6:00 p.m. the night before and then started the next morning. The first half day and the last day of the fast were definitely the hardest to endure. The second day, I was so busy that I didn't even notice, and hunger was almost non-existent.

- The slight headache I had during the whole fast was worse on the third day, and I got a little dizzy a few times. I figured out later that I should have been getting some salt and potassium. I think if I would have supplemented with homemade mineral water, or a buffered electrolyte such as Succeed S! Caps, these symptoms would have been more manageable.

- Since I didn't want to be in the kitchen during the fast, I should have made foods for after the fast before I started. I didn't do that and was scrambling for correct choices on that third evening.

- Blood-glucose and ketone readings were interesting. I had higher blood-glucose readings and lower ketones in the morning, which I attribute to gluconeogenesis.[82] I almost wanted to keep going just to see how high the afternoon ketones would get.

- I learned that you shouldn't finish a three-day fast with a large meal. First, the digestive system will protest noticeably. Second, eating a high number of calories all at once sent my ketones down and blood glucose up. So go slow when reintroducing food after your fast. And don't forget to drink lots of water to stay hydrated. This will also help reduce blood-sugar readings.

7

. . .

Customizing Your Diet

Following a ketogenic diet involves knowing what to eat and how much to eat within the parameters of the diet. The goal of a ketogenic diet plan is to determine how many calories you need to maintain or achieve your ideal body weight, and then figure out the right amount of fat, protein and carbohydrate to eat within that calorie limit. This result should help you get to or maintain your ideal weight while also achieving nutritional ketosis.

In this chapter, I'll present the step-by-step method I've developed to help your build your own customized ketogenic diet. It relies on an exchange system of choices for selecting foods that have the correct amount of fat, protein and carbohydrate. This should help make it easier for you to implement the diet. First, let's get an overview of the step-by-step process we wil use. This will take into account your individual physical characteristics and needs.

1. Establish the ideal weight that you want to reach or maintain. This can be the weight at which you feel best, or it can be from a chart.
2. Figure out how many calories you need to eat to maintain your ideal weight.
3. Use your ideal weight and caloric intake to determine how many grams of fat, protein and carbohydrate to eat on a daily basis.
4. Use macronutrient gram amounts to figure out which foods to eat in the proper portions.

Now we'll walk through a hypothetical example for a fictitious woman named Sue Diets. You'll see specific instructions on how to complete the steps, which appendixes to use and how to work out the simple formulas. You can then apply that information with your individual characteristics to create your own custom plan.

Step-By-Step Directions

Now that we have an overview of the process, let's walk through a hypothetical example, using an individual's physical characteristics to customize a ketogenic diet for our friend Sue Diets. I've made up a sample worksheet for Sue at the end of this section.

> Sue Diets is a 32-year-old female who is five foot six and weighs 150 pounds. Her job is sedentary, but she walks a mile three times a week. She would like to use a ketogenic diet to provide some protection against a cancer reoccurrence, and she would also like to take off 10 pounds. She feels her ideal weight is 140 pounds.

Step 1: Determine your ideal body weight.

Use your height to determine the applicable ideal weight range using the table in appendix C, and then select your ideal weight target.

> Sue goes to appendix C, and looks up the ideal weight range that matches her height. She writes the range on her copy of the Macronutrient Worksheet provided in appendix F. She then decides on her ideal weight.

- Sue's height: 5'6"
- Ideal Weight Range from appendix C: 117–143 pounds
- Ideal Weight: 140 pounds

Step 2: Establish your daily calorie requirement to maintain ideal body weight.

Using one of the calorie calculator websites listed below, enter your ideal weight and activity level to determine the daily calorie amount you should consume to maintain a normal body mass index (BMI). Alternatively, use the formulas in appendix D to establish your ideal weight.

- http://www.cimedicalcenter.com/metabolism-p124
- http://www.bcm.edu/cnrc/caloriesneed.cfm

> Sue uses one of the links above to find her ideal weight (also shown in appendix D). Using an online calculator, she obtains results which show she can eat approximately 1700 calories per day to reach and maintain her ideal weight of 140 pounds.

> (Note on BMI Measurement: Choose an ideal weight target that results in a BMI in the normal weight category. A BMI around 22 falls in the middle of that category and is a recommended target.)

Sue notes that the BMI given on the calculator for her ideal weight is 22.6, so 140 pounds is a good ideal-weight target for her.

Step 3: Use ideal body weight and daily caloric intake to create macronutrient targets.

Use the tables in appendix E to determine your total daily intake of fat, protein and carbohydrate (macronutrients) in the correct proportions.

Now that Sue knows her calorie limit is 1700, and her ideal weight is 140 pounds, she can now use the tables in appendix E to determine how much fat, protein and carbohydrate she can have each day. The amount of fat, protein and carbs in her diet are known as the ketogenic macronutrient levels or KML. To establish her KML, Sue goes to appendix E and finds the table for the 1600–1700 calorie range and reads the 140 pound line.

Sue's KML results are shown in the table below. Protein amounts are shown first because they are the foundation upon which the other macronutrient amounts are based. Consuming the correct amount of daily protein will help Sue maintain her muscle mass while she gets to her ideal weight of 140 pounds. The carb levels are static at the start of the diet and set at 12 grams to facilitate ketosis. The fat-gram levels simply make up the remainder of the 1700 calories she is allowed. The following information is taken from appendix E:

Ideal weight (pounds)	Ideal weight (Kg)	Protein grams	Protein calories	Carb grams	Carb calories	Fats for 1700 calories/day	
						Fat g	Fat cal
140	64	64	256	12	48	155	1396

(Note that when you are calculating food exchanges, you must use grams, not calories. This is because the caloric value of protein foods won't give accurate counts because they also contain fat.)

Knowing that she must use grams to calculate exchanges, Sue then writes her macronutrient gram levels on the Macronutrient Worksheet, as shown below:

Section 2: Total daily macronutrient amounts based on ideal weight

Using appendix E, find your macronutrient levels based on your ideal weight and daily calorie target

Ideal weight	Protein amount per day	Net carbs per day	Fat amount per day
	Protein grams	Net carb grams	Fat grams
140	64	12	155

Step 4: Use your macronutrient amounts to choose foods in the correct proportions.

Determine your number of macronutrient exchanges by converting the macronutrient grams to exchanges.

With a caloric target of 1700, Sue now knows she can have the following amounts of macronutrients on a daily basis:

- 64 grams of protein
- 12 grams of carbohydrate
- 155 grams of fat

Sue converts these gram measurements into "exchange" units using the following formulas and records them on her Macronutrient Worksheet.

- Each lean protein exchange averages about 7 grams of protein. Sue divides 7 grams into her allowance of 64 grams. She can have 9 protein exchanges per day.
- Each fat and oil exchange is equal to about 12 grams of fat. Her fat allowance is 155 grams so she divides that by 12. She can have about 13 fat exchanges each day.
- Net carbs are counted in total grams. She can choose foods that add up to 12 net carbs each day.

Section 2: Total daily macronutrient amounts based on ideal weight

Using appendix E, find your macronutrient levels based on your ideal weight and daily calorie target.			
Ideal weight	Protein amount per day	Net carbs per day	Fat amount per day
	Protein grams	Net carb grams	Fat grams
140	64	12	155
Number of daily exchanges:	9	12	13

On the next page, I've included Sue's completed Macronutrient Worksheet.

Macronutrient Worksheet: Sample for Sue Diets

Use appendixes C, D, and E to complete this tracking sheet. Choose your calorie target. In section 2, write down the total grams of each macronutrient from the tables in appendix E. Then divide the total protein and fat grams allowed each day by the macronutrient exchange values shown below. You can then see how many exchanges of each macronutrient you can have each day.

Section 1: Use appendixes C and D to find your ideal weight and calorie targets

Height: ____*5'6"*____ Ideal weight range (appendix C): _____*117-143*_____

Ideal weight target: _____*140*_____

Daily calories to reach ideal weight target (appendix D): _____*1699*_____

Daily calorie target: _____*1700*_____

Macronutrient Exchange Values

For the food exchange lists in appendix G, these are the basic gram/calorie breakdowns. Divide your macronutrient allowances by these numbers to get your exchanges:

- Each protein exchange has about 7 grams of protein.
- Each fat exchange has about 12 grams of fat.
- For carbohydrates, calculate net carbs.

Section 2: Total daily macronutrient amounts based on ideal weight

Using appendix E, find your macronutrient levels based on your ideal weight and daily calorie target.			
Ideal weight	Protein amount per day	Net carbs per day	Fat amount per day
	Protein grams (divide by 7)	Net carb grams (count totals)	Fat grams (divide by 12)
140	*64*	*12*	*155*
Number of daily exchanges:	*9*	*12*	*13*

Now that you know how much of each macronutrient to have at each meal, you can go to the food exchange lists in appendix G and choose the foods you would like to match the exchanges allowed.

Using the Food Exchange Lists

Sue can now go to the Food Exchange lists in appendix G and pick out the foods she wants to eat that match the macronutrient amounts for the day. (She could also use a food-counter book or an online food-tracking database to choose her foods by matching up grams allowed to the amounts associated with each food choice.)

Sue makes a copy of the Exchange Record and Food Diary in appendix H and has her breakfast on Day 1. She has 2 slices of bacon and 2 eggs, and cooks them in 2 tablespoons of butter. She looks at the Food Exchange Lists and finds butter under Fats and Oils and finds bacon and eggs under High Protein Moderate Fats. She notes that 1 tablespoon of butter is one fat exchange; 2 slices of bacon are 1 fat exchange, 1 protein exchange and 2 net carbs; and each egg counts as 0.5 of a fat exchange and 1 protein exchange:

Fat and Oil Foods

	Calories	Fat (g)	Carbs (g)	Fiber (g)	Net carbs	Protein (g)
Butter, 1 tbsp.	100	12	0	0	0	0

High-Protein Moderate-Fat Foods

	Calories	Fat (g)	Carbs (g)	Fiber (g)	Net carbs	Protein (g)
Bacon, cooked, 2 slices«	92	9	2	0	2	4
Egg, whole, large, plain, 1 ea.	72	5	0	0	0	6

On her tracking sheet, she writes down what she ate and fills in the appropriate boxes for a total of 4 fat exchanges and 3 protein exchanges. She also counts 2 net carbs for the bacon.

Food	Fat Exchange	Protein Exchange	Net Carbs
Butter, 2 tbsp.	2	0	0
Bacon, 2 slices	1	1	2
Eggs, 2 ea.	1	2	0
Total	4	3	2

Why Use Exchanges?

The idea of exchanges is to make it simple to determine how much of each macronutrient you can have each day, without resorting to constant mathematical calculations involving food weight and caloric value. But as you might imagine, nothing is ever simple. You'll note that net carbs must be included for the bacon consumed as part of Sue's breakfast. Since carb restriction is so very important, in the Food Exchange Lists in appendix G you'll find a « symbol associated with fat and protein foods that also contain "stray" net carbs. Count them up and fill in one box on the tracking sheet for each net carb consumed.

A similar complexity is involved when eating foods like nuts and cheeses that contain a combination of protein, fat and carbohydrate. To help minimize the difficulty in tracking stray protein and fat grams, detailed food lists with gram counts are provided to help distinguish more clearly how many exchanges should be counted for each portion of a "combination food." As a general rule, 0.5 is the smallest exchange unit counted. Here's how the Food Exchange Lists are organized:

- Fat and Oil Foods
- High-Fat Moderate-Protein Combination Foods
- High-Fat Low-Protein Combination Foods
- High-Protein Moderate-Fat Combination Foods
- Fat-Protein-Carb Combination Foods
- Lean-Protein Foods
- Carbohydrate Foods
- Miscellaneous Foods

For your convenience, I've also provided an alphabetically arranged Food Exchange List that includes the fat and protein exchanges and the net carb grams for the same foods as listed in the eight categories above.

Meal Exchanges

Over time, you'll find that there are certain meals you tend to repeat. Instead of going back to the Food Exchange lists to find the proper exchanges for repeat meals, I've created a Meal Exchange Log in appendix I to help you record whole meals and their exchange values. Here's an example log entry for the bacon-and-eggs breakfast discussed above:

Meal description	Fat exchanges	Protein exchanges	Net carbs
Bacon and eggs breakfast: 2 poached eggs, 1 tablespoon butter, 2 slices bacon	4	3	2

This log will come in handy if you're a creature of habit. Even if you aren't, you'll probably find the Meal Exchange Log useful for familiarizing yourself with exchange values and recording them consistently.

You might create a separate Meal Exchange Log for the meals you expect to eat throughout each day: breakfast, lunch, dinner, snack. Add new meals and their exchange values to the appropriate log as you go along. This will allow you to build a handy meal reference. As an example, just turn to your breakfast meal log and select a meal you'd like to repeat and, voilà, all your exchange data is available, no need to look up each item again.

As a final note, if you find that this exchange system doesn't work for you, you can use a website such as Fitday.com to track total grams of fat, protein, and carb. This method works great for tracking total gram counts of each macronutrient. The only drawback is that you cannot choose specific amounts of macronutrients. You can only assign percentages in increments of 5%. Cronometer.com may be easier to use, since it offers a ketogenic-diet setting.

Tips on Using Your Customized Ketogenic Diet Plan

- Try not to eat all of your macronutrients at one meal. Eating large amounts of food in one sitting will spike blood sugar and insulin. The goal for blood glucose is low and steady.

- If you like to have smaller and more frequent meals, you may want to divide your carbs up between only a couple of meals, and then have no carbs during the other meals. Otherwise, it becomes challenging to stick to such small carb allowances at each meal.

- If the foods you like aren't on the Food Exchange Lists, you can use an online food-tracking program or a food-counts book that provides carb, protein, and fat gram counts for foods. (See the Tips to Help You Start and Succeed section in chapter 5 for product suggestions.)

- Mix and match food choices as you wish, as long as you stay within the macronutrient levels for your ideal weight.

- Pay attention to tracking your choices correctly. Some food choices will count as a protein and fat or a combination of protein, fat, and carb. Remember that carbs have to be counted as net grams, whether they are consumed as part of a fat or protein food, or consumed as a food from the Carbohydrate Foods list.

- One way to implement the diet with consistency is to carefully create meals and record them on Meal Exchange Logs with one log assigned for each meal throughout the day: breakfast, lunch, dinner and snack. This will allow you to record total exchanges for meals you expect to prepare repeatedly. After you have perhaps a dozen meals documented on a log, it will be easy to mix and match them to provide a variety of foods without having to research the exchanges again. Also, think outside the box. Eggs and bacon can be eaten at lunch or dinner, and steak with vegetables makes a great breakfast.

- It will probably be easier if you start by selecting "food units" instead of preparing complex meals that require measuring multiple ingredients. Eating foods that are easily measured in units can make it simple to identify and track their exchange values. Examples of food units would include: eggs, avocados, sausage links, bacon strips, pats of butter, prepackaged chunks of cheese, shrimp, and hamburger patties.

8

...

Ketogenic Cooking Techniques

Ketogenic diet cooking is all about creating meals from fresh, basic ingredients. Each meal should be based on a protein source of meat, poultry or seafood, prepared and dressed with natural fats such as butter, olive oil or coconut oil. Low-carb vegetables and salads with dressings complement the meal. Sauces and dressings are all made of natural fats and added as you like. I work from the premise that sauces and dressings are the key to taking a ketogenic meal from okay to fabulous.

Although most ketogenic meals are simple and straighforward, there is a challenge in preparing more complex foods such as stews. The trick is to substitute new keto-friendly cooking techniques for traditional cooking methods. For instance, stews and chili usually start out with coating the meat in flour. For a ketogenic stew, the flour is eliminated. To thicken stew near the end of the cooking process, some of the cooked vegetables are pureed with some of the liquid and then returned to the pot to make a thicker final product. Another way to thicken stews and sauces is to cook them longer over low heat to reduce some of the liquid.

Meats, poultry and seafood choices should be prepared using the following methods: roasting, grilling, poaching, baking, sautéing, broiling and steaming. No flour, breading or cracker crumbs should be used, as they add carbohydrates.

The same goes for cooking vegetables. All of the methods mentioned above will work for vegetables as well. Cooking vegetables in water (boiling instead of steaming) can destroy vitamins and leach minerals, but if you are making a stew, at least some of vitamins and minerals are recovered because the cooking water becomes part of the final meal.

Below I offer some useful tips, techniques and tools for creating ketogenic meals when time is short, and a list of snack ideas which are delicious and relatively easy to prepare. I also include a list of my go-to cookbooks and recipe websites.

Time-Saving Cooking Tips

If time is short during the week, there are ways to stay on track:

- Cook all your food for the coming week on the weekend.
- Roast a chicken, debone it, and make part of it into chicken salad.
- Bake a beef or pork shoulder, and slice it for easy snacks.
- Make egg salad, tuna salad and other meat salads; these are easy and fast.
- Prepare vegetable casseroles for a quick side-dish option.
- Slow-cook stews or beef chili, and freeze them in single-serving containers.
- Make hollandaise, pesto and other fat-based sauces and dressings. Store them in the refrigerator so you can grab a quick spoonful for baked fish or meat.
- Find local sources with low-carb food offerings. A local deli may have chicken salads, baked fish and other low-carb choices. Or look for specialty restaurants that have meat kabobs or chef salads you can buy on the run.
- Stock the cupboard and refrigerator with easy-to-fix, low-carb foods: canned tuna and chicken, sardines, or hard-boiled eggs for egg salad. A mixture of mayonnaise and cream cheese makes a great dressing for tuna or chicken salad. Mayonnaise and melted butter mixed together really tastes great on egg salad.
- If you cook in the evening, make extra servings and store them for the next meal.
- Learn new, efficient ways to cook. For instance, lay out bacon on a cookie sheet, and bake it in the oven. It's a lot faster and less messy than frying it in a skillet.

Quick Ketogenic Snack Ideas

These snack ideas do include some cheese in small amounts. I think this is acceptable on an occasional basis.

- Lunch meat roll-ups: spread a slice of ham, turkey or salami with cream cheese or mayonnaise, roll it up by itself or roll it in a lettuce leaf.
- Leftover meat from dinner: steak tips, pork chunks, chicken cut into bite-sized pieces mixed with butter, sour cream or avocado.
- Hard-boiled eggs, sliced and spread with mayonnaise or sour cream.
- Smoked salmon strips spread with softened cream cheese. Add dill and lemon juice for another flavor.
- Beef jerky cured without sugar. The People's Choice brand has some sugar free options that are very good.

- Tuna mixed with mayonnaise and piled on cucumber rounds.
- Olives stuffed with feta cheese.
- Roasted nuts, except for cashews.
- Several dill pickles.
- Pork rinds dipped in a mixture of sour cream and low-carb salsa.
- Pork rinds dipped in ranch dressing or pesto sauce.
- Jicama, radish, or turnip sticks with full-fat sour-cream dip or ranch dressing.
- Baked chicken wings (no breading) and blue-cheese dip.
- Antipasto dish: salami/prosciutto, olives, small amounts of cheese.
- Celery stuffed with a cream-cheese/blue-cheese mixture.
- Celery stuffed with cream cheese mixed with minced olives.
- Celery stuffed with cream cheese mixed with curry or any other spice you like.
- Macadamia nuts fried in butter and sprinkled with cinnamon.

Useful Kitchen Supplies

These supplies are indispensable for making your life easier while on a ketogenic diet. In particular, I use a nonstick skillet, food scale, spatulas, and parchment paper almost daily.

- Heat-resistant silicone spatulas for scraping all fat from cookware. (Small ones work great for scooping up salad dressing from the bottom of a bowl.)
- Digital food scale with ounce and gram measurements.
- Travel cooler and freezer packs for bringing food to work or on leisure activities.
- Small plastic containers with snap-on lids with silicone seals.
- Small wire whisks to incorporate oils into a sauce or dressing.
- Handheld immersion blender.
- Parchment paper for baking.
- Nonstick frying pans.
- Silicone muffin pans and cookie-sheet liners.
- Food processor.
- Glass measuring cups in 2-, 4- and 8-cup sizes.
- Ceramic quiche pan or deep-dish pie plate.
- Single-serving glass bowls with plastic lids.
- Krups egg cooker. (Amy Berger says this is the best $30 you'll ever spend.)

Recipe Resources

The following recipe sites are useful as a guide. A ketogenic diet for cancer therapy may restrict some of the foods used in these recipes, so make modifications as needed. Typing "low-carb recipes" in Google or another search engine will provide more sites with recipes to peruse as well.

- http://www.atkinsforseizures.com/
- http://www.ketogenic-diet-resource.com/low-carb-recipes.html
- http://www.charliefoundation.org/resources-tools/resources-2/find-recipes
- http://ketonutrition.blogspot.ca/#!/2012/10/keto-recipes-and-foods.html
- http://www.atkins.com/Recipes.aspx
- http://site.matthewsfriends.org/
- http://borum.ifas.ufl.edu/ketogator/MealMaking.html
- http://www.genaw.com/lowcarb/
- http://www.yourlighterside.com
- Here's a great post on baking with coconut flour: http://comfybelly.com/2012/06/baking-with-coconut-flour-2/
- And another post on cooking with almond flour: http://comfybelly.com/2009/01/baking-with-almond-flour/

Recommended Cookbooks

These books provide more ideas for meal planning and include techniques for preparing foods. Not all of the recipes are specifically ketogenic, but they should help generate ideas for variety in your meals.

- *The Keto Cookbook* by Dawn Martenz: This book was written by the mother of a child with epilepsy. I have both the Kindle and paperback version and found the paperback version much easier to use.
- *500 Low-Carb Recipes* by Dana Carpender. This goes in and out of print.
- *300 15-Minute Low-Carb Recipes* by Dana Carpender.
- *Eating Stella Style* by George Stella.
- *George Stella's Livin' Low Carb* by George Stella and Cory Williamson.
- *New Atkins for a New You: The Ultimate Diet for Shedding Weight and Feeling Great* by Drs. Eric Westman, Jeff Volek, and Stephen Phinney.

- *Fat Fast Cookbook* by Dana Carpender.
- *Paleo Cooking* by Elana Amsterdam. Great recipes for dairy-free, low-carb breads in this book.

In addition, most whole-food recipes from your favorite cookbook can be adapted to a low-carb, ketogenic version.

9

...

Dining Out on a Ketogenic Diet

Many people want to know if they can eat at restaurants while on a ketogenic diet. The short answer is yes! You can enjoy dining out while on a ketogenic diet provided that you are careful about what you order. Being on this diet will not prevent you from experiencing a nice meal with friends and family. Don't be shy about customizing your order and asking for substitutions when necessary. As people become more health conscious and as food allergies become more common, waitstaff are not put off by special requests. Here is a guide, provided courtesy of nutritionist Amy Berger, to help you select appropriate foods that will allow you to continue getting the benefits of your unique diet.

General Tips

Choose simply prepared dishes: grilled, baked, or roasted meats, poultry, seafood, and non-starchy vegetables and salads. Avoid all pasta, rice, bread, potatoes, corn, beans, soda, and desserts (including fruit). Small amounts of cheese with various meals, such as fajitas or salads, are okay.

Tips for Specific Cuisines

- *Mexican:* Fajitas are a great choice; ask the server not to bring the tortillas, and ask for extra vegetables instead of beans and/or rice. Fajita fillings are just grilled meat and vegetables, and you can enjoy sour cream, small amounts of cheese, guacamole, and pico de gallo as condiments. Be sure there's no corn in the pico de gallo. (At Chipotle, you can get meat, lettuce and vegetables in a bowl rather than in a tortilla wrap.)

- *Middle Eastern/Greek:* Choose kebabs or other grilled-meat dishes. Ask for extra vegetables or meat instead of rice or pita bread. Avoid hummus, stuffed grape leaves (they usually contain rice), anything with beans, and high-starch foods such as potatoes.

- *Chinese/Japanese:* Ask for your dishes to be steamed or prepared with no sauce. (Sauces typically contain sugar and corn starch.) Use soy sauce or hot mustard as a condiment. Great choices for Chinese takeout are steamed chicken or shrimp with mixed vegetables. Some restaurants also offer grilled chicken/beef on skewers. Avoid rice, noodles, wontons, dumplings, deep-fried foods, and tempura (due to the breading). Sashimi is wonderful; avoid sushi rice.

- *Italian:* Pasta is obviously not permitted, but most Italian restaurants have many other options that are suitable for a very low-carbohydrate diet. Choose salads, steaks, chicken, pork, or seafood with vegetables. Avoid bread and breadsticks, and ask for no croutons on your salad. Ask for extra non-starchy green leafy vegetables as side dishes instead of pasta or potatoes.

- *Diner/American Bistro:* These restaurants usually have a very diverse menu, and finding suitable options will be easy. Just use the same logic as for anywhere else: no grain or other starchy carbohydrates and no sweets for dessert. Fantastic choices are cobb, chef, or Caesar salads (no croutons!) with full-fat dressing. Perfectly fine choices are bunless hamburgers or breadless sandwiches. Always ask for non-starchy vegetables (like greens) instead of fries or other potato sides. You can often substitute a simple house salad for a starchy side dish. Other good selections include any type of roasted meat, chicken, fish, or a platter of egg or tuna salad on a bed of lettuce.

- *Breakfast:* Stick with eggs, bacon, ham, and sausage. Avoid pancakes, waffles, potatoes, toast, bagels, muffins, fruit, juice, and jam or jelly. Western omelets are a great option (eggs, ham, onion, peppers) as are any type of omelet that contains eggs, meat, cheese, and/or low-starch veggies (peppers, spinach, mushrooms, onions, zucchini). Any other eggs are great, too: poached, scrambled, over-easy, or hard-boiled. Avoid bottled ketchup, which contains high-fructose corn syrup (HFCS). Use mustard, mayonnaise, and hot sauce as condiments.

- *Salads:* Customize your salad as necessary: no dried cranberries, fruit, or crunchy noodles. Stick with lettuce, spinach, and other greens. Suitable additions are chopped hard-boiled egg, bacon, cheese, avocado, ham, turkey, chicken, steak, salmon, olives, cucumbers, sliced peppers, radishes, and other non-starchy vegetables. Use oil and vinegar or a high-fat dressing like ranch or blue cheese. Avoid thousand island, French, honey mustard, raspberry vinaigrette, and other sweetened dressings. (Besides olive oil, you can use avocado or macadamia oil to make delicious homemade vinaigrettes.)

- *Chain restaurants:* You can find suitable choices at chain restaurants like Applebee's, Chili's, Olive Garden, and Outback Steakhouse. Just ask for the appropriate substitutions. For example, at Outback, ask for double broccoli instead of a potato, and avoid the bread they bring as an appetizer.

Beware of Hidden Dining Pitfalls

Restaurant staff use many different techniques to prepare and present food. Sugar is often added to enhance flavors. Don't be shy about asking your server for details on how foods are prepared. For instance, some restaurants add flour or pancake batter to their eggs to make omelets fluffier. Ask if this is the case, and, if so, ask if they'll prepare your eggs without other additives. (Or stick with hard-boiled, poached, over-easy or sunny-side-up eggs.)

- If there is a sauce with ingredients you're not sure of, ask the server to tell you what's in it. Many sauces contain sugar, corn syrup, corn starch, and/or flour. It's best to stay with simply prepared dishes to avoid this.

- Be careful with condiments. As mentioned above, ketchup is loaded with HFCS, and many salad dressings are high in sugar and corn syrup. Your best bets for condiments (if you need them at all) are mustard (any kind except honey mustard), mayonnaise, melted butter, olive oil, macadamia oil, and vinegar (white, red wine, apple cider).

- Full-fat, low-carbohydrate salad dressings are also permitted. Look at labels in supermarkets to get an idea of which types are best. The carb count per two-tablespoon serving should be two grams or less.

- Prepare yourself ahead of time! Most restaurants have their menus posted online. Look in advance to see what will be suitable for you so you'll have an easier time ordering. Suggest a change of location if necessary.

Travel Tips

Traveling can make staying on an eating program difficult. The tips from Miriam Kalamian below should help you stay on track.

Automobile

- Pack a cooler with small plastic containers of your favorite meals. You are less likely to stray from your plan if you have familiar foods at hand.

- Bring water, and stay well hydrated!

Air Travel

- Carry small packages of nuts and individually wrapped cheese sticks.

- Choose salads with protein (chicken, boiled egg, deli ham, sliced cheese) at the airport. Choose salad dressings with the least amount of carbs per serving. Look for mayonnaise packets to use with the protein. You can also eat chilled butter pats to get the fats you need.

- Pack nuts and protein powder in plastic sandwich bags.

- If you're checking a bag, you can bring your favorite (unopened) salad dressing and a jar of olives. If you want to take MCT oil, pour it into an aluminum water bottle with a leak proof cap. Triple bag this in plastic and add a note explaining what it is (TSA may want to know). Bring clean plastic bags for the return trip.

Conferences

- Breakfast: Stick to scrambled/boiled eggs, with bacon or sausage or cheese. Eat chilled butter pats for extra fat. Ask for half-and-half or heavy cream instead of milk or creamer.

- Lunch: Choose deli meats, tuna, or chicken salad. Scrap the bread and double the salad veggies (minus carrots). Look for olive oil and vinegar (avoid balsamic).

- Dinner: Cut the protein food in half. Ask your waiter to wrap the extra piece. Choose grilled veggies, no sauces. Add olive oil and/or butter. Make sure you get all the oils from the bottom of the plate or bowl.

- Snack: Macadamia nuts are perfect! You may also want to bring individually wrapped cheddar cheese cubes or sticks.

Social Events

- Bring your own meal or eat before you arrive. It's difficult to fight off the "please, just have one bite" or "but I made this just for you" comments if you are hungry or don't have an alternative.

10

...

Other Factors and Resources

The following information covers various topics that may answer questions from readers and provide related information that might be helpful.

What about Exercise?

Gentle physical activity increases well-being. Whenever possible, get up and get moving! Keep it light though. When muscles are overtaxed (working them past the point of having enough oxygen to do the work), lactic acid builds up in muscle tissue. This lactic acid can be recycled into glucose via a biochemical process called the Cori cycle, and this can provide fuel for cancer cells. Go easy and choose mild aerobic exercise such as walking instead of jogging. (Gentle walking after a meal may direct glucose to muscles instead of to tumor tissue.) Lift light weights instead of doing heavy weight training.

Alcohol Consumption

Straight spirits and dry red wines are optional while on a ketogenic diet. Moderation and self-experimentation are essential, as alcohol can have a greater, faster effect while in ketosis. Individuals will need to monitor and assess the effects of alcohol on their blood-glucose and ketone levels and adjust intake accordingly. Some individuals have indicated that a glass of dry red wine has very little effect on blood glucose, and "vino therapy," as one individual so eloquently put it, is an important part of a relaxation strategy.

Stress

Stress can be a confounding factor for achieving target levels of blood glucose because it affects hormones that can increase blood-glucose levels. When we are "stressed out," the body releases many types of "flight or fight" hormones that drive up blood-glucose and insulin levels. While it is unrealistic to expect to avoid stress, it's a good idea to minimize external causes of stress, and find some relaxation techniques to help reduce it and its effects. Yoga, meditation, craftwork, listening to music and gardening are all good forms of relaxation techniques.

Illness, Medications and Menstrual Cycles

Getting sick with a cold or the flu often results in higher levels of blood glucose. In addition, most cold medications are laced with some type of sugar. It's a good idea to search out cold and flu medication that is carb free and stock up. Ask your pharmacist to assist you. Women should be aware that the onset of menstruation also elevates blood glucose for a few days.

Sick Days

Nausea and vomiting are common in people receiving chemotherapy. You may want to review the research on short-term fasting. If you do chose to eat during chemo days, you may want to reduce the amount of fat in your meals.

Diarrhea can be a complication of certain cancers (colon and pancreatic cancer and lymphoma). It can also result from chemotherapy, radiation, and malabsorption. Talk to your medical team about your options.

Flu viruses may cause vomiting and diarrhea, which can quickly lead to dehydration and the loss of electrolytes. Keep well hydrated. Sucking on ice chips can help. Salted broth is an excellent option if tolerated. If vomiting and diarrhea continue, Beth Zupec-Kania[83] of the Charlie Foundation suggests this homemade mineral water remedy:

- ½ tsp of baking soda
- ½ tsp Morton Lite salt
- 4 cups water
- Dissolve salts in water, drink 1 cup every 2 hours

You can also use stevia-sweetened "sports drinks" that contain sodium and other electrolytes. When you are able to eat again, choose bland foods that smell good to you and are palatable. Some good choices include avocado, cheese, and coconut milk. Ease back into fats/oils with mayonnaise, coconut oil, or MCT. Keep meals small.

Until you are back on your feet, you should test blood glucose frequently. If it drops below 55 mg/dL (3 mmol/L), consider sipping on one to two tablespoons of apple or orange juice.

How Long Should I Stay on the Diet?

Diet duration is a tough question to answer. I believe a change in eating habits should be a permanent change so that the benefits are also permanent. However, we don't have any science-based data on this, so it really depends on individual responses to the diet. Some people have found that when they discontinued the diet, their cancer markers worsened, and, in some cases, the cancer returned. Others have been able to resume a less restrictive diet (but still low carb) without that happening. If you experience success using the diet for treating your cancer, and your cancer markers are negative (meaning no evidence of cancer), you might decide to move to a diet that includes a larger selection of foods. If so, I would advise you to keep a close eye on cancer-marker test results over time.

Concerns about Acidity and Alkalinity

Many people have asked me about cancer-treatment diets that focus on the consumption of more alkaline foods to combat the acidity of cancer. Here is the conclusion I have come to after having conversations with scientists who are doing research on the effects of a ketogenic diet and conducting my own research.

As I have discussed, cancer cells have defective mitochondria and defective energy-making processes, termed collectively as oxidative phosphorylation. To compensate, cancer cells use a basic energy process called glycolysis or compensatory fermentation. This fermentation process creates a byproduct called lactate. Fermentation is similar to the process that muscles use when they work too hard without enough oxygen: there's a buildup of lactic acid, and this causes pain in the muscle. Lactic acid is, as you can guess, acidic. Hence, the acidity associated with cancer is a downstream consequence of the cancer cells' metabolic dysfunction, not of the kinds of food being eaten. As ketogenic expert Dr. Dominic D'Agostino explained to me, "An alkaline diet can't hurt, but it won't do much to restore defective cancer-cell metabolism or even change the tumor microenvironment."

A ketogenic diet has a much more powerful effect on overriding the metabolic dysfunction of cancer than eating more alkaline foods could ever have. As has been explained, a ketogenic diet limits carbohydrate, protein, and, if needed, calories, and this lowers blood-glucose and insulin levels. The lack of fuel puts metabolic pressure on cancer cells. In contrast, adding alkaline foods to the diet means adding more vegetables and fruits. This adds more carbohydrate to the diet, especially with the consumption of fruit, which increases blood glucose and which, in turn, gives the cancer cells the fuel they need to grow.

Finally, I believe the reason alkaline diets have been successful for some people is that they are so low in calories that they induce ketosis, especially for people who are already underweight or not insulin-resistant.

Antioxidants

An additional point on the acid/alkaline debate is that of antioxidants. As previously mentioned, one of the ways that cancer cells avoid normal cellular apoptosis (a process by which cells commit suicide when they are damaged) is by using great amounts of glucose to repair free-radical damage. When glucose is limited, they are more likely to succumb to the constant free-radical bombardment with which all cells contend. The idea behind the use of antioxidants is to help normal cells fight free radicals. But in the case of cancer cells, the goal is to actually kill the cancer cell by increasing free-radical damage. Radiation therapy is designed to do just this by overwhelming cancer cells with free radicals.

Although the conventional viewpoint is that vegetables, fruit and supplements (vitamins C and E) in large amounts are cancer suppressing, these foods also provide large amounts of antioxidants (molecules which neutralize free radicals). It's possible that cancer cells could use these antioxidant molecules to fight off free radicals and increase their chances of survival. At least one study has reported that taking anti-oxidants results in accelerated cancer progression.[84] However, the science is by no means settled on this issue. But it is possible that antioxidants may not be as helpful as we think.

Ketogenic Diet and Vegetarianism

Recommendations for treating cancer with a ketogenic diet call for a very low carbo-hydrate intake of less than 12 grams per day, with the goal of reducing blood-glucose and insulin levels. Generally, for most people, eating a moderate amount of protein and staying below an intake of 50 grams of carbohydrate per day results in ketosis.

However, adhering to a vegetarian diet that restricts animal fats and proteins nec-essarily requires eating more carbohydrate. This higher carb intake has the effect of increasing baseline blood glucose and short circuiting ketosis.

There is very little research or guidance available on eating a vegetarian or vegan ketogenic diet. However, a book called *New Atkins for a New You: The Ultimate Diet for Shedding Weight and Feeling Great* by Dr. Eric Westman, Dr. Jeff Volek and Dr. Ste-phen Phinney has a vegetarian section that may be helpful, as does the Atkins website. As stated on the Atkins website, the recommendations of carb intake for vegetarians start at 30 net carbs per day. This is generally workable for weight loss and mild ketosis, but may be too high for the ketogenic diet cancer treatment.

Having said that, any reduction in carbohydrate intake should help to lower blood-glucose and insulin levels, which is generally helpful for fighting inflammation and changing the metabolic environment so that it is more hostile to cancer cells. Here are some resources on the web that may help with a vegetarian or vegan low-carb diet:

- http://www.sheknows.com/food-and-recipes/articles/4408/ stocking-the-low-carb-vegetarian-kitchen

- http://lowcarbdiets.about.com/od/vegetarian/a/veganlowcarb.htm

- http://www.healthcentral.com/diabetes/c/17/20763/ lowcarb-vegetarian/2?ic=2601

Resources for More Information

The following websites provide more information about ketogenic diets:

- Dr. Dominic D'Agostino's website: www.ketonutrition.blogspot.com

- Dietary Therapies, Miriam Kalamian's website: www.dietarytherapies.com

- Patricia Daly's website: www.patriciadaly.com

- Dr. Colin Champ's blog: www.cavemandoctor.com

- The Charlie Foundation: www.charliefoundation.org

- Matthew's Friends: www.matthewsfriends.org

- The Ketogenic Diet Center at Johns Hopkins Hospital in Baltimore, MD: http://www.hopkinsmedicine.org/neurology_neurosurgery/specialty_areas/ epilepsy/pediatric_epilepsy/ketogenic_diet.html

- Jimmy Moore's podcast with Dr. Thomas Seyfried: http:// www.thelivinlowcarbshow.com/shownotes/1172/ dr-thomas-seyfried-on-killer-carbs-ketosis-as-a-cancer-cure-episode-302/

- Dr. Thomas Seyfried's lecture at the Ancestral Health Symposium 2012: http:// www.youtube.com/watch?v=sBjnWfT8HbQ

- Dr. Eugene Fine's lecture at the Ancestral Health Symposium 2012: http://www. youtube.com/watch?v=04A5U6IlHqk

- What You Need to Know about Cancer and Metabolic Control Analysis, an interview with Dr. Thomas Seyfried on Robb Wolf's Paleo Crossfit podcast: http://www.crossfit.com/cf-journal/seyfriedInterview.pdf

- The Townsend Letter's review of Dr. Seyfried's book *Cancer as Metabolic Disease: On the Origin, Management, and Prevention of Cancer*: http://www.townsendletter.com/Dec2012/warcancer1212.html
- Adrienne C. Scheck, PhD, has done work with ketogenic diets and cancer at the Barrow Institute: http://www.thebarrow.org/Research/Neuro_Oncology/213930

These are some of the books I use as references:

- *Get Started with the Ketogenic Diet for Cancer: A Step-by-Step Guide to Implementation* by Miriam Kalamian. Available on her website: dietarytherapies.com. Miriam has a new book coming out in the Fall of 2017 through Chelsea Green Publishing. Her new book is titled *Keto for Cancer: The Ketogenic Diet as a Targeted Nutritional Strategy: A Guide for Patients and Practitioners based on the Metabolic Theory of Cancer.*

- *Cancer as Metabolic Disease: On the Origin, Management, and Prevention of Cancer* by Thomas N. Seyfried, PhD.

- *Ketogenic Diets, fifth edition,* by John Freeman, MD, Eric Kossoff, MD, Zahava Turner, RD, and James Rubenstein, MD.

- *Dietary Treatment of Epilepsy: Practical Implementation of Ketogenic Therapy* by Elizabeth Neal, RD.

- *New Atkins for a New You: The Ultimate Diet for Shedding Weight and Feeling Great* by Eric Westman, MD, Jeff Volek, PhD, RD, and Stephen Phinney, MD, PhD.

- *The Art and Science of Low Carbohydrate Living: An Expert's Guide to Making the Life-Saving Benefits of Carbohydrate Restriction Sustainable and Enjoyable* by Jeff Volek, PhD, RD, and Stephen Phinney, MD, PhD.

- *The Art and Science of Low Carbohydrate Performance* by Jeff Volek, PhD, RD, and Stephen Phinney, MD, PhD.

- *The Ketogenic Kitchen* by Patricia Daly and Domini Kemp.

Appendixes

Appendix A: Recommended Supplements

Look for supplements with the lowest carbohydrate levels. Remember, sugar free is not the same as carbohydrate free. Read labels to rule out those that contain sugar alcohols or other hidden carbohydrates. The following supplements are recommended:

- A low-carb multivitamin/mineral supplement. Make sure it contains no more than 100% of the RDA for all micronutrients and that it also contains selenium and zinc. The Nature's Life Mighty Mini Vite Micro Tablet product offers just the minimal baseline and is recommended.

- Vitamin D3 in the form of cholecalciferol, 2000 IU. Country Life makes a gel-cap product made with medium-chain triglycerides.

- Nordic Naturals omega-3 fish oil, 1-2 capsules daily to provide essential fatty acids. Note: fish oil has an anticoagulant effect so it should be discontinued two weeks prior to surgery.

- Magnesium citrate or magnesium glycinate, 400 mg daily, taken at bedtime if possible. Note that if you have kidney problems, you should not take oral magnesium supplements without consulting the physician responsible for treating your kidney issues.

- CoQ10 (Ubiquinol or Ubiquinone), 100 mg daily.

- CardiaSalt, Lite Salt or NuSalt. You can find these salt substitutes at most grocery stores or on Amazon. You can use regular salt or these salt substitutes for flavoring your food.

- Now brand potassium chloride powder. It is very important to get enough potassium each day. Include green vegetables, small amounts of nuts, and avocadoes in your diet on a regular basis. You can also drink homemade mineral water (recipe below).

Homemade mineral water recipe

Follow this recipe exactly, and sip this water only if you have symptoms such as fatigue, dizziness or headaches.

- To one quart of cold water, add exactly one-quarter teaspoon of Now brand potassium chloride powder and exactly one level teaspoon of table or sea salt (provides sodium and chloride). Mix well and store in the refrigerator.

Appendix B: Recommended Health Professionals

Below is a list of recommended health-care professionals who have experience monitoring progress on a ketogenic diet. I know some of these people personally but not all. Please be aware that their availability and services are subject to change.

Health Professionals in the United States of America

Miriam Kalamian, EdM, MS, CNS

Miriam and I maintain an ongoing collaboration with the goal of providing information and tools that people need to successfully implement a ketogenic diet for cancer. She has been a driver in the keto-for-cancer world since 2007 when she first learned that the diet might benefit her own son, Raffi. Miriam draws on her vast experience to answer specific questions and develop personalized diet prescriptions. Miriam also has a book titled *Get Started with the Ketogenic Diet for Cancer: A Step-by-Step Guide to Implementation*, which I recommend you purchase as well to benefit from her vast experience. Miriam has a new book coming out in the Fall of 2017 through Chelsea Green Publishing. It is titled *Keto for Cancer: The Ketogenic Diet as a Targeted Nutritional Strategy: A Guide for Patients and Practitioners based on the Metabolic Theory of Cancer.*
Email: mkalamian@gmail.com
Website: www.dietarytherapies.com

Denise Potter, RD, CSP, CDE

Ms. Potter is an expert in the implementation of ketogenic diets for cancer, epilepsy, diabetes and various other medical conditions. She is a certified diabetes educator and specialist in pediatrics. You can contact her via her website.
Website: http://www.potterketogenic.diet/

Nasha Winters, ND, FABNO, LAC, DIPLOM

Nasha Winters is a naturopathic doctor specializing in the field of oncology. Winters aims to support the whole person via Hippocrates' credo: "Let food be thy medicine."
Optimal Terrain Consulting, Durango, CO. Consultations via phone or Skype
Phone: (970) 403-5409
Email: support@optimalterrainconsulting.com
Website: www.optimalterrainconsulting.com

Jess Higgins Kelley, MNT

Oncology Nutrition Therapist
Nutrition Therapy Institute
Phone: (970) 903-9271 (cell)
Email: jesshkelley@icloud.com
Website: www.remissionnutrition.com

Sarah Barts, MA, RD, CSO, LD

Manager, Dietary Services
Board Certified Specialist in Oncology Nutrition
Minnesota Oncology, Maplewood Cancer Center
Woodbury Cancer Center, St. Paul Cancer Center
Phone: (612) 720-6475 (cell)
Email: Sarah.Barts@usoncology.com

Thomas Cowan, M.D.

Holistic Family Medicine
661 Chenery Street
San Francisco, CA 94131
Phone: (415) 334-1010
Website: http://fourfoldhealing.com

Helen Gelhot, M.D.

Advanced Wellness
12855 N 40 Dr., N Tower, Ste 200, Walker Medical Building
St. Louis, MO 63141
Phone: (314) 576-0094 Skype: htgelhot
Email: MD@advancedwellnessSTL.com
Website: www.advancedwellnessSTL.com

Nathan Goodyear, MD, FAARM

Seasons of Farragut
10607 Deerbrook Drive
Knoxville, TN 37922
Phone: (865) 675-9355
Email: office@seasonswellness.com
Website: www.seasonswellness.com

The Charlie Foundation for Ketogenic Therapies

515 Ocean Ave., #602N
Santa Monica, CA 90402
Phone: (310) 393-2347
Website: https: //www.charliefoundation.org/
Beth Zupec Kania, Consultant Nutritionist
Email: ketogenicseminars@wi.rr.com

Kara Fitzgerald, ND

27 Glen Road
Sandy Hook, CT 06482
Phone: (203) 304-9502
Email: info@drkarafitzgerald.com
Website: http://www.drkarafitzgerald.com/

Ian D. Bier, N.D., Ph.D., L.Ac., FABNO

Human Nature Natural Health
155 Borthwick Avenue, W#102
Portsmouth, NH 03801
Phone: 603-610-7778
Email: info@humannaturenaturalhealth.com
Website: http://www.humannaturenaturalhealth.com/oncology/Ketogenic

Mark O'Neal Speight, MD

Center For Wellness
1258 Mann Drive
Suite 100
Matthews, NC 28105
Phone: (704) 847-2022
Email: centerforwellness@gmail.com
Website: http://www.cfwellness.com/

George Yu, MD

Aegis Medical and Research Associates
Clinical professor of Urology
George Washington University
Washington, DC

Email: George.yu8@gmail.com
Website: http://yufoundation.org/about-us

Mark Renneker, MD

Assistant Clinical Professor
Department of Family and Community Medicine,
University of California, San Francisco
Phone: 415-681-5357
Email: mark.renneker@ucsf.edu
Dr. Renneker specializes in patient advocacy and may be able to point you to other physicians who offer direct patient care.

Health Professionals in the United Kingdom

Dr. Damien Downing

New Medicine Group 144 Harley St
London W1G 7LE
Phone: 0845 67 69 699
Email: damien@newmedicinegroup.com
Website: http://newmedicinegroup.com/practitioners/dr-damien-downing/

Anne Pemberton Bsc(Hon), RGN, PGCE(autism), DipION

Nurse/Nutritional Therapist, EFT practitioner, Metabolic Balance Coach
Galtres House, Lysander Close
York YO30 3XB UK
01904 691591
Email: enq@naltd.co.uk
Also, Email Anne Pemberton: annepem@nutrimed.co.uk
Tel mobile: 07986735118
Website: Nutrition Associates http://www.naltd.co.uk

Matthew's Friends

Emma Williams founded Matthew's Friends, a British organization that promotes the use of ketogenic diets for treating epilepsy. The dietitians on staff may be a resource in the UK.
Website: http://www.matthewsfriends.org/

Health Professionals in Ireland

Patricia Daly, BA Hons, dipNT, mBANT, mNTOI, ITEC

Patricia is a qualified nutritional therapist based in Dublin (Ireland), specializing in the area of integrative cancer care. She has followed a ketogenic diet for over a year now to fight her eye cancer; she has learned a lot in this process and is keen to pass on her knowledge and expertise to her clients. She is also the author of *The Ketogenic Kitchen*, a book on ketogenic cooking with she co-authored with Domini Kemp. Patricia offers phone/Skype consultations for clients.
Website: http://www.patriciadaly.com

Other Ideas for Finding Support

Consider physicians with experience in using the ketogenic diet for epilepsy and who may be able to also assist in cancer cases. The website address below may be helpful.

- http://www.epilepsy.com/epilepsy/keto_physicians

Another idea is to check with the integrative physicians in your area. They are more likely to embrace alternative therapies.

Appendix C: Suggested Ideal Weight Ranges

Using your gender and height, find your suggested weight range. Adjust to your individual needs. If you feel best at 140, but your range is lower, choose the weight at which you feel best.

Men*		Women*	
Height	Ideal Weight	Height	Ideal Weight
4' 10"	85–103 lbs.	4' 10"	81–99 lbs.
4' 11"	90–110 lbs.	4' 11"	86–105 lbs.
5' 0"	95–117 lbs.	5' 0"	90–110 lbs.
5' 1"	101–123 lbs.	5' 1"	95–116 lbs.
5' 2"	106–130 lbs.	5' 2"	99–121 lbs.
5' 3"	112–136 lbs.	5' 3"	104–127 lbs.
5' 4"	117–143 lbs.	5' 4"	108–132 lbs.
5' 5"	122–150 lbs.	5' 5"	113–138 lbs.
5' 6"	128–156 lbs.	5' 6"	117–143 lbs.
5' 7"	133–163 lbs.	5' 7"	122–149 lbs.
5' 8"	139–169 lbs.	5' 8"	126–154 lbs.
5' 9"	144–176 lbs.	5' 9"	131–160 lbs.
5' 10"	149–183 lbs.	5' 10"	135–165 lbs.
5' 11"	155–189 lbs.	5' 11"	140–171 lbs.
6' 0"	160–196 lbs.	6' 0"	144–176 lbs.
6' 1"	166–202 lbs.	6' 1"	149–182 lbs.
6' 2"	171–209 lbs.	6' 2"	153–187 lbs.
6' 3"	176–216 lbs.	6' 3"	158–193 lbs.
6' 4"	182–222 lbs.	6' 4"	162–198 lbs.
6' 5"	187–229 lbs.	6' 5"	167–204 lbs.
6' 6"	193–235 lbs.	6' 6"	171–209 lbs.
6' 7"	198–242 lbs.	6' 7"	176–215 lbs.
6' 8"	203–249 lbs.	6' 8"	180–220 lbs.
6' 9"	209–255 lbs.	6' 9"	185–226 lbs.
6' 10"	214–262 lbs.	6' 10"	189–231 lbs.
6' 11"	220–268 lbs.	6' 11"	194–237 lbs.
7' 0"	225–275 lbs.	7' 0"	198–242 lbs.

Source: http://www.rush.edu/rumc/page-1108048103230.html
* To calculate weight in kilograms, divide by 2.2.

Appendix D: Daily Calorie Requirements

Figure out your daily calories based on your basal metabolic rate (BMR). Calculate your BMR by using your current weight, height, gender and activity level. You can use one of these online calculators if you don't want to do the math yourself:

- http://www.cimedicalcenter.com/metabolism-p124
- http://www.bcm.edu/cnrc/caloriesneed.cfm

I provide the following for those who are technically minded. The calculators provided at the links above use the same equations.

Calculate Basal Metabolic Rate (Harris-Benedict Equation)

Use the following formulas to figure out your individual BMR:

Women: 655 + (4.35 x weight in pounds) + (4.7 x height in inches) - (4.7 x age in years)

Men: 66 + (6.23 x weight in pounds) + (12.7 x height in inches) - (6.8 x age in years)

- Example: You are 38-year-old woman, who is 5'4" and 142 pounds.
- First, convert your height into inches. 5'4" equals 64 inches.
- Now plug your values into the equation above.
- 655 + (4.35 x 142) + (4.7 x 64) - (4.7 x 38)
- 655 + 617.7 + 300.8 - 178.6 = 1394.9
- Your BMR = 1394.9

Calculate Total Calorie Needs

To get a better sense of how many calories your body uses in any given day, you need to factor in your activity level. To determine your total daily calorie needs, multiply your BMR by the appropriate activity factor, as follows:

- If you are sedentary (little or no exercise): BMR x 1.2
- If you are lightly active (easy exercise/sports 1–3 days/week): BMR x 1.375
- If you are moderately active (moderate exercise/sports 3–5 days/week): BMR x 1.55
- If you are very active (hard exercise/sports 6–7 days a week): BMR x 1.725
- If you are extremely active (very hard exercise/sports and physical job): BMR x 1.9

Continuing with our example, let's assume you are lightly active. Multiply your BMR (1394.9) by the activity level factor of 1.375 = 1917.9875 (round up to 1918 calories). The resulting number (1918) is the total number of calories you would need to maintain your current weight. Now use that number to figure your daily calorie target:

- If you are overweight, you can reduce calorie intake by 500 calories per day to work toward weight loss (1918 - 500=1418 calories per day).
- If you are underweight, add 500 calories to your daily total to work toward weight gain.

Appendix E: Ketogenic Macronutrient Levels

Ketogenic Macronutrient Levels: 1200–1300 Calories

Protein amounts are based on ideal weight (to preserve lean muscle mass); carbohydrate levels are static (to facilitate ketosis); and fat amounts make up the balance of total daily calorie limit.

Ideal weight (pounds)	Ideal weight (Kg)	Protein grams	Protein calories	Net carb grams	Net carb calories	Fats for 1200 calories/day		Fats for 1300 calories/day	
						Fat g	Fat cal	Fat g	Fat cal
100	45	45	180	12	48	108	972	119	1072
105	48	48	192	12	48	107	960	118	1060
110	50	50	200	12	48	106	952	117	1052
115	52	52	208	12	48	105	944	116	1044
120	55	55	220	12	48	104	932	115	1032
125	57	57	228	12	48	103	924	114	1024
130	59	59	236	12	48	102	916	113	1016
135	61	61	244	12	48	101	908	112	1008
140	64	64	256	12	48	100	896	111	996
145	66	66	264	12	48	99	888	110	988
150	68	68	272	12	48	98	880	109	980
155	70	70	280	12	48	97	872	108	972
160	73	73	292	12	48	96	860	107	960
165	75	75	300	12	48	95	852	106	952
170	77	77	308	12	48	94	844	105	944
175	80	80	320	12	48	92	832	104	932
180	82	82	328	12	48	92	824	103	924
185	84	84	336	12	48	91	816	102	916
190	86	86	344	12	48	90	808	101	908
195	89	89	356	12	48	88	796	100	896
200	91	91	364	12	48	88	788	99	888
205	93	93	372	12	48	87	780	98	880
210	95	95	380	12	48	86	772	97	872
215	98	98	392	12	48	84	760	96	860
220	100	100	400	12	48	84	752	95	852
225	102	102	408	12	48	83	744	94	844
230	105	105	420	12	48	81	732	92	832
235	107	107	428	12	48	80	724	92	824
240	109	109	436	12	48	80	716	91	816
245	111	110	440	12	48	79	712	90	812
250	114	111	444	12	48	79	708	90	808
255	116	112	448	12	48	78	704	89	804
260	118	113	452	12	48	78	700	89	800
265	120	114	456	12	48	77	696	88	796
270	123	115	460	12	48	77	692	88	792
275	125	116	464	12	48	76	688	88	788
280	127	117	468	12	48	76	684	87	784
285	130	118	472	12	48	76	680	87	780
290	132	119	476	12	48	75	676	86	776
295	134	120	480	12	48	75	672	86	772
300	136	121	484	12	48	74	668	85	768
305	139	122	488	12	48	74	664	85	764
310	141	123	492	12	48	73	660	84	760
315	143	124	496	12	48	73	656	84	756
320	145	125	500	12	48	72	652	84	752
325	148	126	504	12	48	72	648	83	744

Ketogenic Macronutrient Levels: 1400–1500 Calories

Protein amounts are based on ideal weight (to preserve lean muscle mass); carbohydrate levels are static (to facilitate ketosis); and fat amounts make up the balance of total daily calorie limit.

Ideal weight (pounds)	Ideal weight (Kg)	Protein grams	Protein calories	Net carb grams	Net carb calories	Fats for 1400 calories/day		Fats for 1500 calories/day	
						Fat g	Fat cal	Fat g	Fat cal
100	45	45	180	12	48	130	1172	141	1272
105	48	48	192	12	48	129	1160	140	1260
110	50	50	200	12	48	128	1152	139	1252
115	52	52	208	12	48	127	1144	138	1244
120	55	55	220	12	48	126	1132	137	1232
125	57	57	228	12	48	125	1124	136	1224
130	59	59	236	12	48	124	1116	135	1216
135	61	61	244	12	48	123	1108	134	1208
140	64	64	256	12	48	122	1096	133	1196
145	66	66	264	12	48	121	1088	132	1188
150	68	68	272	12	48	120	1080	131	1180
155	70	70	280	12	48	119	1072	130	1172
160	73	73	292	12	48	118	1060	129	1160
165	75	75	300	12	48	117	1052	128	1152
170	77	77	308	12	48	116	1044	127	1144
175	80	80	320	12	48	115	1032	126	1132
180	82	82	328	12	48	114	1024	125	1124
185	84	84	336	12	48	113	1016	124	1116
190	86	86	344	12	48	112	1008	123	1108
195	89	89	356	12	48	111	996	122	1096
200	91	91	364	12	48	110	988	121	1088
205	93	93	372	12	48	109	980	120	1080
210	95	95	380	12	48	108	972	119	1072
215	98	98	392	12	48	107	960	118	1060
220	100	100	400	12	48	106	952	117	1052
225	102	102	408	12	48	105	944	116	1044
230	105	105	420	12	48	104	932	115	1032
235	107	107	428	12	48	103	924	114	1024
240	109	109	436	12	48	102	916	113	1016
245	111	110	440	12	48	101	912	112	1012
250	114	111	444	12	48	101	908	112	1008
255	116	112	448	12	48	100	904	112	1004
260	118	113	452	12	48	100	900	111	1000
265	120	114	456	12	48	100	896	111	996
270	123	115	460	12	48	99	892	110	992
275	125	116	464	12	48	99	888	110	988
280	127	117	468	12	48	98	884	109	984
285	130	118	472	12	48	98	880	109	980
290	132	119	476	12	48	97	876	108	976
295	134	120	480	12	48	97	872	108	972
300	136	121	484	12	48	96	868	108	968
305	139	122	488	12	48	96	864	107	964
310	141	123	492	12	48	96	860	107	960
315	143	124	496	12	48	95	856	106	956
320	145	125	500	12	48	95	852	106	952
325	148	126	504	12	48	94	848	105	948
330	150	127	508	12	48	94	844	105	944
335	152	128	512	12	48	93	840	104	940
340	155	129	516	12	48	93	836	104	936
345	157	130	520	12	48	92	832	104	932

Ketogenic Macronutrient Levels: 1600–1700 Calories

Protein amounts are based on ideal weight (to preserve lean muscle mass); carbohydrate levels are static (to facilitate ketosis); and fat amounts make up the balance of total daily calorie limit.

Ideal weight (pounds)	Ideal weight (Kg)	Protein grams	Protein calories	Net carb grams	Net carb calories	Fats for 1600 calories/day		Fats for 1700 calories/day	
						Fat g	Fat cal	Fat g	Fat cal
100	45	45	180	12	48	152	1372	164	1472
105	48	48	192	12	48	151	1360	162	1460
110	50	50	200	12	48	150	1352	161	1452
115	52	52	208	12	48	149	1344	160	1444
120	55	55	220	12	48	148	1332	159	1432
125	57	57	228	12	48	147	1324	158	1424
130	59	59	236	12	48	146	1316	157	1416
135	61	61	244	12	48	145	1308	156	1408
140	64	64	256	12	48	144	1296	155	1396
145	66	66	264	12	48	143	1288	154	1388
150	68	68	272	12	48	142	1280	153	1380
155	70	70	280	12	48	141	1272	152	1372
160	73	73	292	12	48	140	1260	151	1360
165	75	75	300	12	48	139	1252	150	1352
170	77	77	308	12	48	138	1244	149	1344
175	80	80	320	12	48	137	1232	148	1332
180	82	82	328	12	48	136	1224	147	1324
185	84	84	336	12	48	135	1216	146	1316
190	86	86	344	12	48	134	1208	145	1308
195	89	89	356	12	48	133	1196	144	1296
200	91	91	364	12	48	132	1188	143	1288
205	93	93	372	12	48	131	1180	142	1280
210	95	95	380	12	48	130	1172	141	1272
215	98	98	392	12	48	129	1160	140	1260
220	100	100	400	12	48	128	1152	139	1252
225	102	102	408	12	48	127	1144	138	1244
230	105	105	420	12	48	126	1132	137	1232
235	107	107	428	12	48	125	1124	136	1224
240	109	109	436	12	48	124	1116	135	1216
245	111	110	440	12	48	124	1112	135	1212
250	114	111	444	12	48	123	1108	134	1208
255	116	112	448	12	48	123	1104	134	1204
260	118	113	452	12	48	122	1100	133	1200
265	120	114	456	12	48	122	1096	133	1196
270	123	115	460	12	48	121	1092	132	1192
275	125	116	464	12	48	121	1088	132	1188
280	127	117	468	12	48	120	1084	132	1184
285	130	118	472	12	48	120	1080	131	1180
290	132	119	476	12	48	120	1076	131	1176
295	134	120	480	12	48	119	1072	130	1172
300	136	121	484	12	48	119	1068	130	1168
305	139	122	488	12	48	118	1064	129	1164
310	141	123	492	12	48	118	1060	129	1160
315	143	124	496	12	48	117	1056	128	1156
320	145	125	500	12	48	117	1052	128	1152
325	148	126	504	12	48	116	1048	128	1148
330	150	127	508	12	48	116	1044	127	1144
335	152	128	512	12	48	116	1040	127	1140
340	155	129	516	12	48	115	1036	126	1136
345	157	130	520	12	48	115	1032	126	1132

Ketogenic Macronutrient Levels: 1800–1900 Calories

Protein amounts are based on ideal weight (to preserve lean muscle mass); carbohydrate levels are static (to facilitate ketosis); and fat amounts make up the balance of total daily calorie limit.

Ideal weight (pounds)	Ideal weight (Kg)	Protein grams	Protein calories	Net carb grams	Net carb calories	Fats for 1800 calories/day		Fats for 1900 calories/day	
						Fat g	Fat cal	Fat g	Fat cal
100	45	45	180	12	48	175	1572	186	1672
105	48	48	192	12	48	173	1560	184	1660
110	50	50	200	12	48	172	1552	184	1652
115	52	52	208	12	48	172	1544	183	1644
120	55	55	220	12	48	170	1532	181	1632
125	57	57	228	12	48	169	1524	180	1624
130	59	59	236	12	48	168	1516	180	1616
135	61	61	244	12	48	168	1508	179	1608
140	64	64	256	12	48	166	1496	177	1596
145	66	66	264	12	48	165	1488	176	1588
150	68	68	272	12	48	164	1480	176	1580
155	70	70	280	12	48	164	1472	175	1572
160	73	73	292	12	48	162	1460	173	1560
165	75	75	300	12	48	161	1452	172	1552
170	77	77	308	12	48	160	1444	172	1544
175	80	80	320	12	48	159	1432	170	1532
180	82	82	328	12	48	158	1424	169	1524
185	84	84	336	12	48	157	1416	168	1516
190	86	86	344	12	48	156	1408	168	1508
195	89	89	356	12	48	155	1396	166	1496
200	91	91	364	12	48	154	1388	165	1488
205	93	93	372	12	48	153	1380	164	1480
210	95	95	380	12	48	152	1372	164	1472
215	98	98	392	12	48	151	1360	162	1460
220	100	100	400	12	48	150	1352	161	1452
225	102	102	408	12	48	149	1344	160	1444
230	105	105	420	12	48	148	1332	159	1432
235	107	107	428	12	48	147	1324	158	1424
240	109	109	436	12	48	146	1316	157	1416
245	111	110	440	12	48	146	1312	157	1412
250	114	111	444	12	48	145	1308	156	1408
255	116	112	448	12	48	145	1304	156	1404
260	118	113	452	12	48	144	1300	156	1400
265	120	114	456	12	48	144	1296	155	1396
270	123	115	460	12	48	144	1292	155	1392
275	125	116	464	12	48	143	1288	154	1388
280	127	117	468	12	48	143	1284	154	1384
285	130	118	472	12	48	142	1280	153	1380
290	132	119	476	12	48	142	1276	153	1376
295	134	120	480	12	48	141	1272	152	1372
300	136	121	484	12	48	141	1268	152	1368
305	139	122	488	12	48	140	1264	152	1364
310	141	123	492	12	48	140	1260	151	1360
315	143	124	496	12	48	140	1256	151	1356
320	145	125	500	12	48	139	1252	150	1352
325	148	126	504	12	48	139	1248	150	1348
330	150	127	508	12	48	138	1244	149	1344
335	152	128	512	12	48	138	1240	149	1340
340	155	129	516	12	48	137	1236	148	1336
345	157	130	520	12	48	137	1232	148	1332

Ketogenic Macronutrient Levels: 2000–2100 Calories

Protein amounts are based on ideal weight (to preserve lean muscle mass); carbohydrate levels are static (to facilitate ketosis); and fat amounts make up the balance of total daily calorie limit.

Ideal weight (pounds)	Ideal weight (Kg)	Protein grams	Protein calories	Net carb grams	Net carb calories	Fats for 2000 calories/day		Fats for 2100 calories/day	
						Fat g	Fat cal	Fat g	Fat cal
100	45	45	180	12	48	197	1772	208	1872
105	48	48	192	12	48	196	1760	207	1860
110	50	50	200	12	48	195	1752	206	1852
115	52	52	208	12	48	194	1744	205	1844
120	55	55	220	12	48	192	1732	204	1832
125	57	57	228	12	48	192	1724	203	1824
130	59	59	236	12	48	191	1716	202	1816
135	61	61	244	12	48	190	1708	201	1808
140	64	64	256	12	48	188	1696	200	1796
145	66	66	264	12	48	188	1688	199	1788
150	68	68	272	12	48	187	1680	198	1780
155	70	70	280	12	48	186	1672	197	1772
160	73	73	292	12	48	184	1660	196	1760
165	75	75	300	12	48	184	1652	195	1752
170	77	77	308	12	48	183	1644	194	1744
175	80	80	320	12	48	181	1632	192	1732
180	82	82	328	12	48	180	1624	192	1724
185	84	84	336	12	48	180	1616	191	1716
190	86	86	344	12	48	179	1608	190	1708
195	89	89	356	12	48	177	1596	188	1696
200	91	91	364	12	48	176	1588	188	1688
205	93	93	372	12	48	176	1580	187	1680
210	95	95	380	12	48	175	1572	186	1672
215	98	98	392	12	48	173	1560	184	1660
220	100	100	400	12	48	172	1552	184	1652
225	102	102	408	12	48	172	1544	183	1644
230	105	105	420	12	48	170	1532	181	1632
235	107	107	428	12	48	169	1524	180	1624
240	109	109	436	12	48	168	1516	180	1616
245	111	110	440	12	48	168	1512	179	1612
250	114	111	444	12	48	168	1508	179	1608
255	116	112	448	12	48	167	1504	178	1604
260	118	113	452	12	48	167	1500	178	1600
265	120	114	456	12	48	166	1496	177	1596
270	123	115	460	12	48	166	1492	177	1592
275	125	116	464	12	48	165	1488	176	1588
280	127	117	468	12	48	165	1484	176	1584
285	130	118	472	12	48	164	1480	176	1580
290	132	119	476	12	48	164	1476	175	1576
295	134	120	480	12	48	164	1472	175	1572
300	136	121	484	12	48	163	1468	174	1568
305	139	122	488	12	48	163	1464	174	1564
310	141	123	492	12	48	162	1460	173	1560
315	143	124	496	12	48	162	1456	173	1556
320	145	125	500	12	48	161	1452	172	1552
325	148	126	504	12	48	161	1448	172	1548
330	150	127	508	12	48	160	1444	172	1544
335	152	128	512	12	48	160	1440	171	1540
340	155	129	516	12	48	160	1436	171	1536
345	157	130	520	12	48	159	1432	170	1532

Ketogenic Macronutrient Levels: 2200–2300 Calories

Protein amounts are based on ideal weight (to preserve lean muscle mass); carbohydrate levels are static (to facilitate ketosis); and fat amounts make up the balance of total daily calorie limit.

Ideal weight (pounds)	Ideal weight (Kg)	Protein grams	Protein calories	Net carb grams	Net carb calories	Fats for 2200 calories/ day		Fats for 2300 calories/ day	
						Fat g	Fat cal	Fat g	Fat cal
100	45	45	180	12	48	219	1972	230	2072
105	48	48	192	12	48	218	1960	229	2060
110	50	50	200	12	48	217	1952	228	2052
115	52	52	208	12	48	216	1944	227	2044
120	55	55	220	12	48	215	1932	226	2032
125	57	57	228	12	48	214	1924	225	2024
130	59	59	236	12	48	213	1916	224	2016
135	61	61	244	12	48	212	1908	223	2008
140	64	64	256	12	48	211	1896	222	1996
145	66	66	264	12	48	210	1888	221	1988
150	68	68	272	12	48	209	1880	220	1980
155	70	70	280	12	48	208	1872	219	1972
160	73	73	292	12	48	207	1860	218	1960
165	75	75	300	12	48	206	1852	217	1952
170	77	77	308	12	48	205	1844	216	1944
175	80	80	320	12	48	204	1832	215	1932
180	82	82	328	12	48	203	1824	214	1924
185	84	84	336	12	48	202	1816	213	1916
190	86	86	344	12	48	201	1808	212	1908
195	89	89	356	12	48	200	1796	211	1896
200	91	91	364	12	48	199	1788	210	1888
205	93	93	372	12	48	198	1780	209	1880
210	95	95	380	12	48	197	1772	208	1872
215	98	98	392	12	48	196	1760	207	1860
220	100	100	400	12	48	195	1752	206	1852
225	102	102	408	12	48	194	1744	205	1844
230	105	105	420	12	48	192	1732	204	1832
235	107	107	428	12	48	192	1724	203	1824
240	109	109	436	12	48	191	1716	202	1816
245	111	110	440	12	48	190	1712	201	1812
250	114	111	444	12	48	190	1708	201	1808
255	116	112	448	12	48	189	1704	200	1804
260	118	113	452	12	48	189	1700	200	1800
265	120	114	456	12	48	188	1696	200	1796
270	123	115	460	12	48	188	1692	199	1792
275	125	116	464	12	48	188	1688	199	1788
280	127	117	468	12	48	187	1684	198	1784
285	130	118	472	12	48	187	1680	198	1780
290	132	119	476	12	48	186	1676	197	1776
295	134	120	480	12	48	186	1672	197	1772
300	136	121	484	12	48	185	1668	196	1768
305	139	122	488	12	48	185	1664	196	1764
310	141	123	492	12	48	184	1660	196	1760
315	143	124	496	12	48	184	1656	195	1756
320	145	125	500	12	48	184	1652	195	1752
325	148	126	504	12	48	183	1648	194	1748
330	150	127	508	12	48	183	1644	194	1744
335	152	128	512	12	48	182	1640	193	1740
340	155	129	516	12	48	182	1636	193	1736
345	157	130	520	12	48	181	1632	192	1732

Ketogenic Macronutrient Levels: 2400–2500 Calories

Protein amounts are based on ideal weight (to preserve lean muscle mass); carbohydrate levels are static (to facilitate ketosis); and fat amounts make up the balance of total daily calorie limit.

Ideal weight (pounds)	Ideal weight (Kg)	Protein grams	Protein calories	Net carb grams	Net carb calories	Fats for 2400 calories/day		Fats for 2500 Calories/Day	
						Fat g	Fat Cal	Fat g	Fat Cal
100	45	45	180	12	48	241	2172	252	2272
105	48	48	192	12	48	240	2160	251	2260
110	50	50	200	12	48	239	2152	250	2252
115	52	52	208	12	48	238	2144	249	2244
120	55	55	220	12	48	237	2132	248	2232
125	57	57	228	12	48	236	2124	247	2224
130	59	59	236	12	48	235	2116	246	2216
135	61	61	244	12	48	234	2108	245	2208
140	64	64	256	12	48	233	2096	244	2196
145	66	66	264	12	48	232	2088	243	2188
150	68	68	272	12	48	231	2080	242	2180
155	70	70	280	12	48	230	2072	241	2172
160	73	73	292	12	48	229	2060	240	2160
165	75	75	300	12	48	228	2052	239	2152
170	77	77	308	12	48	227	2044	238	2144
175	80	80	320	12	48	226	2032	237	2132
180	82	82	328	12	48	225	2024	236	2124
185	84	84	336	12	48	224	2016	235	2116
190	86	86	344	12	48	223	2008	234	2108
195	89	89	356	12	48	222	1996	233	2096
200	91	91	364	12	48	221	1988	232	2088
205	93	93	372	12	48	220	1980	231	2080
210	95	95	380	12	48	219	1972	230	2072
215	98	98	392	12	48	218	1960	229	2060
220	100	100	400	12	48	217	1952	228	2052
225	102	102	408	12	48	216	1944	227	2044
230	105	105	420	12	48	215	1932	226	2032
235	107	107	428	12	48	214	1924	225	2024
240	109	109	436	12	48	213	1916	224	2016
245	111	110	440	12	48	212	1912	224	2012
250	114	111	444	12	48	212	1908	223	2008
255	116	112	448	12	48	212	1904	223	2004
260	118	113	452	12	48	211	1900	222	2000
265	120	114	456	12	48	211	1896	222	1996
270	123	115	460	12	48	210	1892	221	1992
275	125	116	464	12	48	210	1888	221	1988
280	127	117	468	12	48	209	1884	220	1984
285	130	118	472	12	48	209	1880	220	1980
290	132	119	476	12	48	208	1876	220	1976
295	134	120	480	12	48	208	1872	219	1972
300	136	121	484	12	48	208	1868	219	1968
305	139	122	488	12	48	207	1864	218	1964
310	141	123	492	12	48	207	1860	218	1960
315	143	124	496	12	48	206	1856	217	1956
320	145	125	500	12	48	206	1852	217	1952
325	148	126	504	12	48	205	1848	216	1948
330	150	127	508	12	48	205	1844	216	1944
335	152	128	512	12	48	204	1840	216	1940
340	155	129	516	12	48	204	1836	215	1936
345	157	130	520	12	48	204	1832	215	1932

Ketogenic Macronutrient Levels: 2600–2700 Calories

Protein amounts are based on ideal weight (to preserve lean muscle mass), carbohydrate levels are static (to facilitate ketosis) and fat amounts make up the balance of total daily calorie limit.

Ideal Weight (pounds)	Ideal Weight (Kg)	Protein grams	Protein calories	Net Carb grams	Net Carb calories	Fats for 2600 Calories/Day		Fats for 2700 Calories/Day	
						Fat g	Fat Cal	Fat g	Fat Cal
100	45	45	180	12	48	264	2372	275	2472
105	48	48	192	12	48	262	2360	273	2460
110	50	50	200	12	48	261	2352	272	2452
115	52	52	208	12	48	260	2344	272	2444
120	55	55	220	12	48	259	2332	270	2432
125	57	57	228	12	48	258	2324	269	2424
130	59	59	236	12	48	257	2316	268	2416
135	61	61	244	12	48	256	2308	268	2408
140	64	64	256	12	48	255	2296	266	2396
145	66	66	264	12	48	254	2288	265	2388
150	68	68	272	12	48	253	2280	264	2380
155	70	70	280	12	48	252	2272	264	2372
160	73	73	292	12	48	251	2260	262	2360
165	75	75	300	12	48	250	2252	261	2352
170	77	77	308	12	48	249	2244	260	2344
175	80	80	320	12	48	248	2232	259	2332
180	82	82	328	12	48	247	2224	258	2324
185	84	84	336	12	48	246	2216	257	2316
190	86	86	344	12	48	245	2208	256	2308
195	89	89	356	12	48	244	2196	255	2296
200	91	91	364	12	48	243	2188	254	2288
205	93	93	372	12	48	242	2180	253	2280
210	95	95	380	12	48	241	2172	252	2272
215	98	98	392	12	48	240	2160	251	2260
220	100	100	400	12	48	239	2152	250	2252
225	102	102	408	12	48	238	2144	249	2244
230	105	105	420	12	48	237	2132	248	2232
235	107	107	428	12	48	236	2124	247	2224
240	109	109	436	12	48	235	2116	246	2216
245	111	110	440	12	48	235	2112	246	2212
250	114	111	444	12	48	234	2108	245	2208
255	116	112	448	12	48	234	2104	245	2204
260	118	113	452	12	48	233	2100	244	2200
265	120	114	456	12	48	233	2096	244	2196
270	123	115	460	12	48	232	2092	244	2192
275	125	116	464	12	48	232	2088	243	2188
280	127	117	468	12	48	232	2084	243	2184
285	130	118	472	12	48	231	2080	242	2180
290	132	119	476	12	48	231	2076	242	2176
295	134	120	480	12	48	230	2072	241	2172
300	136	121	484	12	48	230	2068	241	2168
305	139	122	488	12	48	229	2064	240	2164
310	141	123	492	12	48	229	2060	240	2160
315	143	124	496	12	48	228	2056	240	2156
320	145	125	500	12	48	228	2052	239	2152
325	148	126	504	12	48	228	2048	239	2148
330	150	127	508	12	48	227	2044	238	2144
335	152	128	512	12	48	227	2040	238	2140
340	155	129	516	12	48	226	2036	237	2136
345	157	130	520	12	48	226	2032	237	2132

Ketogenic Macronutrient Levels: 2800–2900 Calories

Protein amounts are based on ideal weight (to preserve lean muscle mass), carbohydrate levels are static (to facilitate ketosis) and fat amounts make up the balance of total daily calorie limit.

Ideal Weight (pounds)	Ideal Weight (Kg)	Protein grams	Protein calories	Net Carb grams	Net carb calories	Fats for 2800 calories/day		Fats for 2900 calories/day	
						Fat g	Fat cal	Fat g	Fat cal
100	45	45	180	12	48	286	2572	297	2672
105	48	48	192	12	48	284	2560	296	2660
110	50	50	200	12	48	284	2552	295	2652
115	52	52	208	12	48	283	2544	294	2644
120	55	55	220	12	48	281	2532	292	2632
125	57	57	228	12	48	280	2524	292	2624
130	59	59	236	12	48	280	2516	291	2616
135	61	61	244	12	48	279	2508	290	2608
140	64	64	256	12	48	277	2496	288	2596
145	66	66	264	12	48	276	2488	288	2588
150	68	68	272	12	48	276	2480	287	2580
155	70	70	280	12	48	275	2472	286	2572
160	73	73	292	12	48	273	2460	284	2560
165	75	75	300	12	48	272	2452	284	2552
170	77	77	308	12	48	272	2444	283	2544
175	80	80	320	12	48	270	2432	281	2532
180	82	82	328	12	48	269	2424	280	2524
185	84	84	336	12	48	268	2416	280	2516
190	86	86	344	12	48	268	2408	279	2508
195	89	89	356	12	48	266	2396	277	2496
200	91	91	364	12	48	265	2388	276	2488
205	93	93	372	12	48	264	2380	276	2480
210	95	95	380	12	48	264	2372	275	2472
215	98	98	392	12	48	262	2360	273	2460
220	100	100	400	12	48	261	2352	272	2452
225	102	102	408	12	48	260	2344	272	2444
230	105	105	420	12	48	259	2332	270	2432
235	107	107	428	12	48	258	2324	269	2424
240	109	109	436	12	48	257	2316	268	2416
245	111	110	440	12	48	257	2312	268	2412
250	114	111	444	12	48	256	2308	268	2408
255	116	112	448	12	48	256	2304	267	2404
260	118	113	452	12	48	256	2300	267	2400
265	120	114	456	12	48	255	2296	266	2396
270	123	115	460	12	48	255	2292	266	2392
275	125	116	464	12	48	254	2288	265	2388
280	127	117	468	12	48	254	2284	265	2384
285	130	118	472	12	48	253	2280	264	2380
290	132	119	476	12	48	253	2276	264	2376
295	134	120	480	12	48	252	2272	264	2372
300	136	121	484	12	48	252	2268	263	2368
305	139	122	488	12	48	252	2264	263	2364
310	141	123	492	12	48	251	2260	262	2360
315	143	124	496	12	48	251	2256	262	2356
320	145	125	500	12	48	250	2252	261	2352
325	148	126	504	12	48	250	2248	261	2348
330	150	127	508	12	48	249	2244	260	2344
335	152	128	512	12	48	249	2240	260	2340
340	155	129	516	12	48	248	2236	260	2336
345	157	130	520	12	48	248	2232	259	2332

Ketogenic Macronutrient Levels: 3000–3100 Calories

Protein amounts are based on ideal weight (to preserve lean muscle mass); carbohydrate levels are static (to facilitate ketosis); and fat amounts make up the balance of total daily calorie limit.

Ideal weight (pounds)	Ideal weight (Kg)	Protein grams	Protein calories	Net carb grams	Net carb calories	Fats for 3000 calories/day		Fats for 3100 calories/day	
						Fat g	Fat cal	Fat g	Fat cal
100	45	45	180	12	48	308	2772	319	2872
105	48	48	192	12	48	307	2760	318	2860
110	50	50	200	12	48	306	2752	317	2852
115	52	52	208	12	48	305	2744	316	2844
120	55	55	220	12	48	304	2732	315	2832
125	57	57	228	12	48	303	2724	314	2824
130	59	59	236	12	48	302	2716	313	2816
135	61	61	244	12	48	301	2708	312	2808
140	64	64	256	12	48	300	2696	311	2796
145	66	66	264	12	48	299	2688	310	2788
150	68	68	272	12	48	298	2680	309	2780
155	70	70	280	12	48	297	2672	308	2772
160	73	73	292	12	48	296	2660	307	2760
165	75	75	300	12	48	295	2652	306	2752
170	77	77	308	12	48	294	2644	305	2744
175	80	80	320	12	48	292	2632	304	2732
180	82	82	328	12	48	292	2624	303	2724
185	84	84	336	12	48	291	2616	302	2716
190	86	86	344	12	48	290	2608	301	2708
195	89	89	356	12	48	288	2596	300	2696
200	91	91	364	12	48	288	2588	299	2688
205	93	93	372	12	48	287	2580	298	2680
210	95	95	380	12	48	286	2572	297	2672
215	98	98	392	12	48	284	2560	296	2660
220	100	100	400	12	48	284	2552	295	2652
225	102	102	408	12	48	283	2544	294	2644
230	105	105	420	12	48	281	2532	292	2632
235	107	107	428	12	48	280	2524	292	2624
240	109	109	436	12	48	280	2516	291	2616
245	111	110	440	12	48	279	2512	290	2612
250	114	111	444	12	48	279	2508	290	2608
255	116	112	448	12	48	278	2504	289	2604
260	118	113	452	12	48	278	2500	289	2600
265	120	114	456	12	48	277	2496	288	2596
270	123	115	460	12	48	277	2492	288	2592
275	125	116	464	12	48	276	2488	288	2588
280	127	117	468	12	48	276	2484	287	2584
285	130	118	472	12	48	276	2480	287	2580
290	132	119	476	12	48	275	2476	286	2576
295	134	120	480	12	48	275	2472	286	2572
300	136	121	484	12	48	274	2468	285	2568
305	139	122	488	12	48	274	2464	285	2564
310	141	123	492	12	48	273	2460	284	2560
315	143	124	496	12	48	273	2456	284	2556
320	145	125	500	12	48	272	2452	284	2552
325	148	126	504	12	48	272	2448	283	2548
330	150	127	508	12	48	272	2444	283	2544
335	152	128	512	12	48	271	2440	282	2540
340	155	129	516	12	48	271	2436	282	2536
345	157	130	520	12	48	270	2432	281	2532

Appendix F: Macronutrient Worksheet

Use appendixes C, D, and E to complete this tracking sheet. Choose your calorie target. In section 2, write down the total grams of each macronutrient from the tables in appendix E. Then divide the total protein and fat grams allowed each day by the macronutrient exchange values shown below. You can then see how many exchanges of each macronutrient you can have each day.

Section 1: Use appendixes C and D to find your ideal weight and calorie targets

Height: _____ Ideal weight range (appendix C): _____

Ideal weight target: _____

Daily calories to reach ideal weight target (appendix D): _____

Daily calorie target: _____

Macronutrient Exchange Values

For the food exchange lists in appendix G, these are the basic gram/calorie breakdowns. Divide your macronutrient allowances by these numbers to get your exchanges:

- Each protein exchange has about 7 grams of protein.
- Each fat exchange has about 12 grams of fat.
- For carbohydrates, calculate net carbs.

Section 2: Total daily macronutrient amounts based on ideal weight

Using appendix E, find your macronutrient levels based on your ideal weight and daily calorie target			
Ideal weight	Protein amount per day	Net carbs per day	Fat amount per day
	Protein grams (divide by 7)	Net carb grams (count totals)	Fat grams (divide by 12)
Number of daily exchanges:			

Now that you know how much of each macronutrient to have at each meal, you can go to the food exchange lists in appendix G and choose the foods you would like to match the exchanges allowed.

Appendix G: Food Exchange Lists

The food lists in this appendix are by no means comprehensive, but they should address most of the common foods suitable for a ketogenic diet. There are many online resources available that contain thousands of food listings. I've recommended several in this book. Here are some examples:

- Cronometer.com is my favorite. It offers a ketogenic-diet setting.
- Fitday.com offers both a web-based application and an application that can be downloaded to a PC.
- MyFitnessPal.com, a web-based application, is another good choice, and it's free.
- FatSecret.com is another free website.
- The USDA's free nutrition database can be found at http://ndb.nal.usda.gov/.
- The Atkins.com website also has some tools for tracking progress on a ketogenic-diet plan.

There are also many food-count books on the market:

- *The Calorie King* gets good reviews on Amazon, and it comes in both a paperback and digital edition.
- *The Complete Book of Food Counts*, ninth edition, by Corrine Netzer.
- Dana Carpender's *Carb and Calorie Counter*.

Calculating Exchanges

I've provided extensive information on the food lists. If you prefer to count total grams for all foods, that can be done. You can also count calories if you prefer, but be aware that protein foods usually contain fat as well, so the calorie counts versus total grams won't be as accurate. If you decide to go the "exchange" route, the general rules for calculating exchanges from any foods that you add to these lists are as follows:

- *Fats and oils:* There are about 10–14 grams of fat in a serving, less than 1 carb or 1 gram of protein.
- *Proteins:* There are about 6–9 grams of protein in a serving, and less than 6 grams of fat. If the food contains over 6 grams of fat, add a 0.5 fat exchange as well.

- *Carbohydrates:* Count the total net carbs of the food item. Each net carb counts as one exchange.

- *Combination foods:* If the food contains more than 4 grams of protein or 6 grams of fat in combination with carbs, count the protein as a 0.5 of a protein exchange, and the fat as 0.5 of a fat exchange, and note the total net carbs as well.

The food lists begin on the next page. If you want to have a food that isn't on the lists, just use the key above to figure out the exchanges. I've also provided blank lines at the bottom of each category's table so that you can add the foods you like. I suggest that you make copies of these lists to keep with copies of your Exchange Record and Food Diary form found in appendix H.

Fat and Oil Foods

Count each item as 1 fat exchange.
The « indicates net carb grams that should be counted in daily totals.

	Calories	Fat (g)	Carbs (g)	Fiber (g)	Net carbs	Protein (g)
Avocado oil, 1 tbsp.	124	14	0	0	0	0
Avocado, Haas, 3 oz. «	102	9	7	5	2	2
Bacon fat, 1 tbsp.	116	13	0	0	0	0
Beef tallow, 1 tbsp.	115	13	0	0	0	0
Butter, 1 tbsp.	102	12	0	0	0	0
Chicken fat, 1 tbsp.	115	13	0	0	0	0
Cocoa butter, 1 tbsp.	120	14	0	0	0	0
Coconut oil, 1 tbsp.	117	14	0	0	0	0
Cream cheese (block), 2 tbsp.«	101	10	1	0	1	2
Flaxseed oil, 1 tbsp.	120	14	0	0	0	0
Ghee, 1 tbsp.	112	13	0	0	0	0
Heavy cream, fluid, 2 tbsp.«	103	11	1	0	1	1
Lard, fresh (non-hydrogenated), 1 tbsp.	115	13	0	0	0	0
Macadamia oil, 1 tbsp.	120	14	0	0	0	0
Mayonnaise (full fat), 1 tbsp.«	99	11	1	0	1	0
MCT oil, 1 tbsp.	100	14	0	0	0	0
Olive oil, 1 tbsp.	119	14	0	0	0	0
Red palm oil, 1 tbsp.	120	14	0	0	0	0
Salad dressing, creamy full fat (<2 carb/serving), 1.5 tbsp.«	130	14	1	0	1	1
Sour cream (full fat, no fillers – e.g. Daisy brand), 4 tbsp.«	120	10	2	0	2	2

High-Fat Moderate-Protein Combination Foods

Count each choice as 1.50 fat exchanges and 0.5 protein exchange.
The « indicates net carb grams that should be counted in daily totals.

	Calories	Fat (g)	Carbs (g)	Fiber (g)	Net carbs	Protein (g)
Nuts, Brazil nut, roasted, 1 oz. «	186	19	3	2	1	4
Nuts, hazelnut, 1 oz. «	183	18	5	3	2	4
Nuts, walnut, 1 oz. «	185	18	4	2	2	4
Seeds, chia, 1 oz. «	140	10	12	10	2	4
Seeds, sesame, 1 oz. «	161	14	7	5	2	5

High-Fat Low-Protein Combination Foods

Count each choice as 1.50 fat exchanges.
The « indicates net carb grams that should be counted in daily totals.

	Calories	Fat (g)	Carbs (g)	Fiber (g)	Net carbs	Protein (g)
Coconut butter, 2 tbsp.«	186	18	8	4	4	2
Coconut, dried, unsweetened, 1 oz. «	165	15	6	4	2	3
Nuts, macadamia, roasted, 1 oz. «	203	22	4	3	1	2
Nuts, pecan, roasted, 1 oz. «	201	21	4	3	1	3

High-Protein, Moderate-Fat Foods

Count each item as 0.5 fat exchange and 1 lean protein exchange.
The « indicates net carb grams that should be counted in daily totals.

	Calories	Fat (g)	Carbs (g)	Fiber (g)	Net carbs	Protein (g)
Bacon, cooked, 2 slices «	92	9	2	0	2	4
Beef, ground, 80% lean, cooked, 1 oz.	74	5	0	0	0	7
Cheese, blue, 1 oz.	100	8	1	0	0	6
Cheese, brie, 1 oz.	95	8	0	0	0	6
Cheese, cheddar, natural, 1 oz. «	114	9	0	0	1	7
Cheese, Mexican blend, 1 oz. «	105	9	1	0	1	7
Cheese, Monterey jack, 1 oz. «	106	9	0	0	1	7
Cheese, mozzarella, part skim, 1 oz. «	72	5	1	0	1	7
Cheese, mozzarella, whole milk, 1 oz. «	90	7	1	0	1	6
Cheese, parmesan, hard, 1 oz. «	111	7	1	0	1	10
Cheese, provolone, 1 oz. «	100	8	1	0	1	7
Cheese, ricotta, whole milk, 0.25 cup «	107	8	2	0	2	7
Cheese, Swiss, 1 oz. «	108	8	2	0	2	8
Duck, roasted, skin eaten, 1 oz.	95	8	0	0	0	5
Egg, whole, large, plain, 1 ea.	72	5	0	0	0	6
Lamb, boneless, cooked, 1 oz.	83	6	0	0	0	7
Pork breakfast sausage, no fillers or sugar, cooked, 1.5 oz.	102	9	0	0	0	7
Pork ribs, roasted, plain, 1 oz.	104	8	0	0	0	8
Pork shoulder, roasted, 1 oz.	82	6	0	0	0	7
Yogurt, Greek, full fat, 3.5 oz. «	95	5	4	0	4	9

Fat-Protein-Carb Combination Foods

Count each choice as 1 fat exchange and 1 protein exchange.
The « indicates net carb grams that should be counted in daily totals.

	Calories	Fat (g)	Carbs (g)	Fiber (g)	Net carbs	Protein (g)
Almond meal (flour), 1 oz. «	160	14	6	3	3	6
Cheese, feta, 3 oz. «	120	11	3	1	2	6
Nuts, almond, roasted, 1 oz. «	172	16	5	3	2	6
Nuts, cashew, 1 oz. «	164	14	10	0	10	8
Seeds, flax, 1 oz. «	152	12	8	7	1	6
Seeds, pumpkin, roasted, 1 oz. «	148	12	4	1	3	9
Seeds, sunflower, roasted, 1 oz. «	168	15	6	3	3	6

Lean Protein Foods

Count each choice as 1 protein exchange.
The « indicates that net carb grams should be counted in daily totals.

	Calories	Fat (g)	Carbs (g)	Fiber (g)	Net carbs	Protein (g)
Beef, ground, 92% lean, cooked, 1 oz.	45	2	0	0	0	7
Beef steak, broiled or baked, 1 oz.	71	4	0	0	0	8
Beef, chuck, blade roast, cooked, 1 oz.	75	4	0	0	0	9
Chicken breast, roasted or baked, skin not eaten, 1 oz.	46	1	0	0	0	9
Chicken thigh, roasted, no skin, 1.0 oz.	55	3	0	0	0	7
Clams, fresh, baked, 1 oz. «	39	2	1	0	1	4
Cottage cheese, 1-2%, 0.25 cup«	41	1	2	0	2	7
Crab, king, fresh, steamed, 1.5 oz.	41	0	0	0	0	7.5
Egg whites, raw, large egg, 2 ea.«	34	0	0	0	.5	7
Elk steak, roasted, 1 oz.	41	.5	0	0	0	8.5
Fish fillet (flounder, sole, scrod) no breading, baked, 2 oz.	49	1	0	0	0	8.5
Fish, salmon fresh fillet, 1 oz.	39	1	0	0	0	7

Fish, salmon, canned pink, 1 oz.	39	1	0	0	0	7
Ham, deli-style, lean, 1 oz. «	35	1	1	0	1	5
Ham, smoked, spiral, 1 oz. «	53	3	1	0	1	5
Pork chops, lean, cooked, 1 oz.	57	3	0	0	0	7
Pork roast, loin, cooked, 1 oz.	70	4	0	0	0	8
Scallops, baked or broiled, 1 oz. «	38	1	1	0	1	6
Shrimp, steamed or boiled, 1 oz. «	39	1	0	0	0	8
Tuna, canned, water pack, 1 oz.	33	0	0	0	0	7
Turkey breast, roasted, no skin, 1 oz.	38	0	0	0	0	9
Turkey thigh, roasted, no skin, 1 oz.	52	2	0	0	0	8
Yogurt, Greek, 0% fat, 3 oz. «	50	0	3.5	0	3.5	9

Carbohydrate Foods

Count total net carbs for each choice.
The « indicates that a 0.5 protein exchange should also be counted in daily totals.

	Calories	Fat (g)	Carbs (g)	Fiber (g)	Net carbs	Protein (g)
Asparagus, cooked, 1 cup «	46	2	6	4	2	5
Beans, cooked (black, kidney, chickpeas, lentils) 0.25 cup «	55	0	10	3	7	4
Beans, green, cooked, 1 cup	34	.5	8	4	4	2
Blueberries, raw, whole, 0.25 cup	21	0	5	1	4	0
Broccoli, cooked, chopped, 0.5 cup	27	0	6	3	3	2
Brussel sprouts, raw, 1 cup	38	0	8	3	5	3
Cabbage, green, raw, shredded, 4 oz.	23	0	5	2	3	1
Carrots, baby, raw, 2 oz.	20	0	6	2	4	0
Cauliflower, cooked, 1 cup	28	0	6	2	4	2
Celery, raw, chopped, 1 cup	36	0	7	4	3	2
Cucumber, raw, sliced, 10 oz.	29	0	6	2	4	1
Eggplant, raw, 6 oz.	33	0	8	5	3	1

Garlic, 6 cloves	24	0	6	0	6	0
Green beans, cooked, 0.5 cup	22	0	5	1	4	1
Kale, raw, chopped, 2 oz.	28	0	6	1	5	2
Lemon juice, 1 tbsp.	3	0	1	0	1	0
Lettuce, any green leaf, shredded, 3 cups	24	0	6	3	3	3
Lettuce, iceberg, shredded, 3 cups	24	0	6	3	3	0
Lettuce, romaine shredded, 3 cups	24	0	6	3	3	3
Lime juice, 1 tbsp.	3	0	1	0	1	0
Mushrooms, button, raw, 6 oz. «	37	1	6	2	4	5
Mushrooms, portabella, raw, 4 oz.	29	0	6	2	4	3
Onion, green, 0.5 cup	16	0	4	1	3	1
Onion, white, raw, 0.5 cup	33	0	7	1	6	1
Pepper, bell, raw, 4 oz.	23	0	5	2	3	0
Potato, white, cooked, 0.5 cup	95	4	13	2	11	1
Raspberries, raw, whole, 0.5 cup	32	0	7	4	3	1
Rice, white, cooked, 0.25 cup	51	0	11	0	11	1
Shallots, chopped, 2 tbsp.	14	0	4	0	4	0
Spinach, cooked, from frozen, 5 oz. «	57	3	5	3	2	4
Spinach, raw, 6 oz.	38	1	6	4	2	1
Squash, spaghetti, cooked, 1 cup	75	0	10	2	8	1
Squash, summer, cooked, sliced, 1 cup	36	0	8	3	5	2
Strawberries, raw, whole, 0.5 cup	23	0	6	2	4	0
Swiss chard, chopped coarse, 3 cups	21	0	4	2	2	2
Tomato sauce, 0.5 cup	40	0	8	2	6	2
Tomato, raw, 6 oz.	31	0	7	2	5	1
Turnips, raw, 4 oz.	32	0	7	2	5	1

Note on Spices: add 0.5 carb to your carb totals if over ½ teaspoon is added to meals.

Miscellaneous Foods

Add your choice of foods here. Count total grams for each choice.

Food Description	Calories	Fat (g)	Carbs (g)	Fiber (g)	Net carbs	Protein (g)
Olives, black, 1 cup	141	13	8	4	4	1
Olives, green, 1 cup	193	20	5	4	1	1
Pork rinds, fried, 0.75 oz.	116	7	0	0	0	13*

*Note on pork rinds: The protein in this food is inferior in quality. Count the protein grams but limit amounts eaten so as not to displace other more complete protein foods.

Alphabetical Food Exchange List

Alphabetical food exchange list	Fat exchange	Net carb grams	Protein exchange
Almond meal (flour), 1 oz.	1	3	1
Asparagus, cooked, 1 cup	0	2	½
Avocado oil, 1 tbsp.	1	0	0
Avocado, Haas, 3 oz.	1	2	½
Bacon fat, 1 tbsp.	1	0	0
Bacon, cooked, 2 slices	1	2	½
Beans, cooked (black, kidney, chickpeas, lentils) 0.25 cup	0	7	½
Beans, green, cooked, 1 cup	0	4	½
Beef steak, broiled or baked, 1 oz.	½	0	1
Beef tallow, 1 tbsp.	1	0	0
Beef, chuck, blade roast, cooked, 1 oz.	½	0	1
Beef, ground, 80% lean, cooked, 1 oz.	½	0	1
Beef, ground, 92% lean, cooked, 1 oz.	0	0	1
Blueberries, raw, whole, 0.25 cup	0	4	0
Broccoli, cooked, chopped, 0.5 cup	0	3	0
Brussels sprouts, raw, 1 cup	0	5	0
Butter, 1 tbsp.	1	0	0
Cabbage, green, raw, shredded, 4 oz.	0	3	0
Carrots, baby, raw, 2 oz.	0	4	0
Cauliflower, cooked, 1 cup	0	4	0
Celery, raw, chopped, 1 cup	0	3	0
Cheese, blue, 1 oz.	½	0	1
Cheese, brie, 1 oz.	½	0	1
Cheese, cheddar, natural, 1 oz.	1	1	1
Cheese, feta, 3 oz.	1	2	1
Cheese, Mexican blend, 1 oz.	1	1	1
Cheese, Monterey jack, 1 oz.	1	1	1
Cheese, mozzarella, part skim, 1 oz.	0	1	1
Cheese, mozzarella, whole milk, 1 oz.	½	1	1
Cheese, parmesan, hard, 1 oz.	½	1	1 ½
Cheese, provolone, 1 oz.	½	1	1
Cheese, ricotta, whole milk, 0.25 cup	½	2	1
Cheese, Swiss, 1 oz.	½	2	1

Chicken breast, roasted or baked, skin not eaten, 1 oz.	0	0	1
Chicken fat, 1 tbsp.	1	0	0
Chicken thigh, roasted, no skin, 1 oz.	½	0	1
Clams, fresh, baked, 1 oz.	0	1	½
Cocoa butter, 1 tbsp.	1	0	0
Coconut butter, 2 tbsp.	1 ½	4	0
Coconut oil, 1 tbsp.	1	0	0
Coconut, dried, unsweetened, 1 oz.	1	2	½
Cottage cheese, 1-2%, 0.25 cup	0	2	1
Crab, king, fresh, steamed, 1.5 oz.	0	0	1
Cream cheese (block), 2 tbsp.	1	1	0
Cucumber, raw, sliced, 10 oz.	0	4	0
Duck, roasted, skin eaten, 1 oz.	½	0	½
Egg whites, raw, large egg, 2 ea.	0	0.5	1
Egg, whole, large, plain, 1 ea.	½	0	1
Eggplant, raw, 6 oz.	0	3	0
Elk steak, roasted, 1 oz.	0	0	1
Fish fillet (flounder, sole, scrod) no breading, baked, 2 oz.	0	0	1
Fish, salmon fresh fillet, 1 oz.	0	0	1
Fish, salmon, canned pink, 1 oz.	0	0	1
Flaxseed oil, 1 tbsp.	1	0	0
Garlic, 6 cloves	0	6	0
Ghee, 1 tbsp.	1	0	0
Green beans, cooked, 0.5 cup	0	4	0
Ham, deli style, lean, 1 oz.	0	1	1
Ham, smoked, spiral, 1 oz.	0	1	1
Heavy cream, fluid, 2 tbsp.	1	1	0
Kale, raw, chopped, 2 oz.	0	5	0
Lamb, boneless, cooked, 1 oz.	½	0	1
Lard, fresh (non-hydrogenated), 1 tbsp.	1	0	0
Lemon juice, 1 tbsp.	0	1	0
Lettuce, any green leaf, shredded, 3 cups	0	3	0
Lettuce, iceberg, shredded, 3 cups	0	3	0
Lettuce, romaine shredded, 3 cups	0	3	0
Lime juice, 1 tbsp.	0	1	0
Macadamia oil, 1 tbsp.	1	0	0

Mayonnaise (full fat), 1 tbsp.	1	1	0
MCT oil, 1 tbsp.	1	0	0
Mushrooms, button, raw, 6 oz.	0	4	½
Mushrooms, portabella, raw, 4 oz.	0	4	0
Nuts, almonds, roasted, 1 oz.	1 ½	2	1
Nuts, Brazil nut, roasted, 1 oz.	1 ½	1	½
Nuts, cashew, 1 oz.	1	10	1
Nuts, hazelnuts, 1 oz.	1 ½	2	½
Nuts, macadamia, roasted, 1 oz.	2	1	0
Nuts, pecan, roasted, 1 oz.	2	1	0
Nuts, walnut, 1 oz.	1 ½	2	½
Olive oil, 1 tbsp.	1	0	0
Olives, black, 1 cup	1	4	0
Olives, green, 1 cup	2	1	0
Onion, green, 0.5 cup	0	3	0
Onion, white, raw, 0.5 cup	0	6	0
Pepper, bell, raw, 4 oz.	0	3	0
Pork breakfast sausage, no fillers or sugar, cooked, 1.5 oz.	1	0	1
Pork chops, lean, cooked, 1 oz.	½	0	1
Pork ribs, roasted, plain, 1 oz.	½	0	1
Pork rinds, fried, 0.75 oz.	½	0	2*
Pork roast, loin, cooked, 1 oz.	½	0	1
Pork shoulder, roasted, 1 oz.	½	0	1
Potato, white, cooked, 0.5 cup	½	11	0
Raspberries, raw, whole, 0.5 cup	0	3	0
Red palm oil, 1 tbsp.	1	0	0
Rice, white, cooked, 0.25 cup	0	11	0
Salad dressing, creamy full fat (<2 carb/serving), 1.5 tbsp.	1	1	0
Scallops, baked or broiled, 1 oz.	0	1	1
Seeds, chia, 1 oz.	1	2	½
Seeds, flax, 1 oz.	1	1	1
Seeds, pumpkin, roasted, 1 oz.	1	3	1
Seeds, sesame, 1 oz.	1	2	½
Seeds, sunflower, roasted, 1 oz.	1	3	1
Shallots, chopped, 2 tbsp.	0	4	0
Shrimp, steamed or boiled, 1 oz.	0	0	1

Sour cream (full fat, no fillers – e.g. Daisy brand), 4 tbsp.	1	2	0
Spinach, cooked, from frozen, 5 oz.	½	2	½
Spinach, raw, 6 oz.	0	2	0
Squash, spaghetti, cooked, 1 cup	0	8	0
Squash, summer, cooked, sliced, 1 cup	0	5	0
Strawberries, raw, whole, 0.5 cup	0	4	0
Swiss chard, chopped coarse, 3 cups	0	2	0
Tomato sauce, 0.5 cup	0	6	0
Tomato, raw, 6 oz.	0	5	0
Tuna, canned, water pack, 1 oz.	0	0	1
Turkey breast, roasted, no skin, 1 oz.	0	0	1
Turkey thigh, roasted, no skin, 1 oz.	0	0	1
Turnips, raw, 4 oz.	0	5	0
Yogurt, Greek, 0% fat, 3 oz.	0	3.5	1
Yogurt, Greek, full fat, 3.5 oz.	½	4	1

*Note on pork rinds: The protein in this food is inferior in quality. Count the protein grams but limit amounts eaten so as not to displace other more complete protein foods.

Spice Carb Counts

The listings below show the net carbs in 1 tablespoon of dried spice.

Allspice, ground	3.0		Nutmeg	2.0
Basil, dried	0.9		Onion powder	5.2
Black pepper	2.4		Oregano, ground	0.4
Caraway seed	0.8		Paprika	1.2
Cardamom, ground	2.4		Parsley, dried	0.3
Cayenne pepper	1.6		Peppermint, fresh	0.1
Cinnamon, ground	1.7		Poppy seeds	1.2
Cloves	1.7		Poultry seasoning	2.0
Coriander seed	0.6		Pumpkin pie spice	3.1
Cumin, ground	2.1		Sage, ground	0.4
Curry powder	1.6		Spearmint, dried	0.3
Fennel seed	0.7		Tarragon, ground	2.0
Garlic powder	5.3		Thyme, ground	1.1
Ginger, ground	3.1		Vanilla extract	1.6
Imitation vanilla extract	0.3		White pepper	3.0
Mace, ground	1.6			

Appendix H: Exchange Record and Food Diary

Daily exchange allowances: Fats:_____ Protein:_____ Carbs:_____ Calories:_____

	Day 1	Day 2	Day 3	Day 4	Day 5	Day 6	Day 7
Breakfast							
Lunch							
Dinner							
Snack							
Water	☐☐☐☐☐ ☐☐☐☐☐	☐☐☐☐☐ ☐☐☐☐☐	☐☐☐☐☐ ☐☐☐☐☐	☐☐☐☐☐ ☐☐☐☐☐	☐☐☐☐☐ ☐☐☐☐☐	☐☐☐☐☐ ☐☐☐☐☐	☐☐☐☐☐ ☐☐☐☐☐
Fats (12 grams/ exchange)	☐☐☐☐☐ ☐☐☐☐☐ ☐☐☐☐☐	☐☐☐☐☐ ☐☐☐☐☐ ☐☐☐☐☐	☐☐☐☐☐ ☐☐☐☐☐ ☐☐☐☐☐	☐☐☐☐☐ ☐☐☐☐☐ ☐☐☐☐☐	☐☐☐☐☐ ☐☐☐☐☐ ☐☐☐☐☐	☐☐☐☐☐ ☐☐☐☐☐ ☐☐☐☐☐	☐☐☐☐☐ ☐☐☐☐☐ ☐☐☐☐☐
Protein (7 grams/ exchange)	☐☐☐☐☐ ☐☐☐☐☐ ☐☐☐☐☐	☐☐☐☐☐ ☐☐☐☐☐ ☐☐☐☐☐	☐☐☐☐☐ ☐☐☐☐☐ ☐☐☐☐☐	☐☐☐☐☐ ☐☐☐☐☐ ☐☐☐☐☐	☐☐☐☐☐ ☐☐☐☐☐ ☐☐☐☐☐	☐☐☐☐☐ ☐☐☐☐☐ ☐☐☐☐☐	☐☐☐☐☐ ☐☐☐☐☐ ☐☐☐☐☐
Net carbs (count totals)	☐☐☐☐☐ ☐☐☐☐☐ ☐☐☐☐☐ ☐☐☐☐☐	☐☐☐☐☐ ☐☐☐☐☐ ☐☐☐☐☐ ☐☐☐☐☐	☐☐☐☐☐ ☐☐☐☐☐ ☐☐☐☐☐ ☐☐☐☐☐	☐☐☐☐☐ ☐☐☐☐☐ ☐☐☐☐☐ ☐☐☐☐☐	☐☐☐☐☐ ☐☐☐☐☐ ☐☐☐☐☐ ☐☐☐☐☐	☐☐☐☐☐ ☐☐☐☐☐ ☐☐☐☐☐ ☐☐☐☐☐	☐☐☐☐☐ ☐☐☐☐☐ ☐☐☐☐☐ ☐☐☐☐☐
Ketones							

Appendix I: Meal Exchange Log

Copy and use this form to track total exchanges for meals that you eat more frequently.

Meal description	Fat exchanges	Protein exchanges	Net carbs

Appendix J: Conversions and Measurements

Rules for Measures

- Multiply grams by 0.0353 to get the weight in ounces.
- Multiply ounces by 28.35 to get the weight in grams.

Dry-Measure Equivalents

Measurement	Equal to	Equal to	Equals
3 teaspoons	1 tablespoon	1/2 ounce	14.3 grams
2 tablespoons	1/8 cup	1 ounce	28.3 grams
4 tablespoons	1/4 cup	2 ounces	56.7 grams
5 1/3 tablespoons	1/3 cup	2.6 ounces	75.6 grams
8 tablespoons	1/2 cup	4 ounces	113.4 grams
12 tablespoons	3/4 cup	6 ounces	.375 pound
32 tablespoons	2 cups	16 ounces	1 pound

Volume (Liquid) Measurements

American cups and quarts equal to	American ounces equal to	Metric (milliliters and liters)
2 tbsp.	1 fl. oz.	30 ml
¼ cup	2 fl. oz.	60 ml
½ cup	4 fl. oz.	125 ml
1 cup	8 fl. oz.	250 ml
1 ½ cups	12 fl. oz.	375 ml
2 cups or 1 pint	16 fl. oz.	500 ml
4 cups or 1 quart	32 fl. oz.	1000 ml or 1 liter
1 gallon	128 fl. oz.	4 liters

Oven Temperatures

Fahrenheit	Celsius
250° F	130° C
300° F	150° C
350° F	180° C
400° F	200° C
450° F	230° C

Abbreviations

Abbreviation	Full term
ea.	each
oz.	ounce
tbsp.	tablespoon
tsp.	teaspoon
c	cup

Ketone Conversion Formula

The exact calculation (and easier method) is shown here:

Value in mg/dL divided by 10.41 (easier method divides by 10)	mmol/L
Value in mmol/L multiplied by 10.41 (easier method divides by 10)	mg/dL

Blood Glucose Conversion Formula

The exact calculation is shown here:

Value in mg/dL multiplied by 0.0555	mmol/L
Value in mmol/L multiplied by 18.0182	mg/dL

This is the easier method:

Value in mg/dL divided by 18	mmol/L
Value in mmol/L multiplied by 18	mg/dL

Blood Sugar Conversion Table for G/K Index:

Note that if the blood glucose reading is higher than 115 mg/dL, go to next column set.

Blood glucose mg/dl	Blood glucose mmol	Blood glucose mg/dl	Blood glucose mmol
50	3.0	120	6.7
55	3.1	125	6.9
60	3.3	130	7.2
65	3.6	135	7.5
70	3.9	140	7.8
75	4.2	145	8.1
80	4.4	150	8.3
85	4.7	155	8.6
90	5.0	160	8.9
95	5.3	165	9.2
100	5.6	170	9.4
105	5.8	175	9.7
110	6.1	180	10.0
115	6.4	185	10.3

References

Glossary

Aerobic exercise   Sustained, cadenced exercise that increases your heart rate; also referred to as cardio.

Acidosis   A condition in which the blood is too acidic (blood pH falls below 7.35), which manifests in the symptoms of rapid breathing, confusion or lethargy. It can be fatal if not treated.

Amino acids   The molecular building blocks of proteins. There are over one hundred amino acids, eight are essential, meaning they have to be obtained from the diet.

Antioxidants   Substances that neutralize harmful free radicals and reactive oxygen species (ROS) in the body.

Apoptosis   The metabolic process of programmed cell death. In normal cells, apoptosis is triggered when a cell is damaged, which minimizes toxic releases to surrounding cells. Cancer cells tend to have defective mechanisms, which fail to trigger apoptosis.

Atherosclerosis   Clogging, narrowing, and hardening of blood vessels by plaque deposits.

ATP   Adenosine triphosphate. A molecule that transports chemical energy within cells for metabolic purposes.

Beta cells   Specialized cells in the pancreas that produce the hormone insulin.

Blood lipids   The medical term for the total cholesterol, triglycerides, and HDL and LDL cholesterol in your blood.

Blood pressure   The pressure your blood exerts against the walls of your arteries during a heartbeat.

Blood glucose   The amount of glucose in your bloodstream; also called blood glucose.

Body mass index (BMI)   A measure of body fat based on height and weight for adults.

Branched-chain amino acids (BCAA)   A category of three specific amino acids   isoleucine, leucine and valine. They function in the body to ramp up protein synthesis and provide energy. Leucine, especially, has been show to stimulate tumor growth.

Cancer cachexia   A syndrome of progressive weight loss, lack of appetite, and persistent erosion of muscle mass associated with having cancer.

Carbohydrate (carb)   A carbon- and water-based macronutrient that, when broken down by digestion into simple sugars (such as glucose), provides a source of energy.

Casein   The main protein found in milk and in milk products such as cheese. It has insulin-spiking properties and should be avoided on a ketogenic diet.

Cellular respiration   The process that all cells use to produce energy. It involves both glucose and oxygen and involves cellular mitochondria.

Chemotherapy   A treatment for cancer that uses one or more cell-killing anti-cancer drugs ("chemotherapeutic agents") as part of a standard of care in cancer cases.

Cholesterol   A waxy substance essential for many of the body's functions, including the manufacturing of hormones and making cell membranes.

Compensatory fermentation   An increased dependence on glycolysis (glucose fermentation) in cells with damaged cellular-respiration capabilities.

Cori cycle   The metabolic pathway in which lactic acid is produced by metabolizing glucose without the presence of oxygen. The lactic acid in the muscles moves to the liver and is converted to glucose, which then returns to the muscles and is converted back to lactate.

Diabetes   A group of diseases that result in too much sugar in the blood (high blood glucose). See type 1 diabetes and type 2 diabetes.

Diuretic   A substance that causes fluid to be eliminated from the body by increasing urination.

Essential fatty acids (EFAs)   Two classes of essential dietary fats that must be obtained from food or supplements. The two classes are omega-3 and omega-6, with the numbers designating the location of the first chemical double bond in the molecule.

Essential nutrients   Nutrients that are required for life but which the body cannot make internally. Hence, they must be obtained from the diet.

Fat   One of the three macronutrients; an organic compound that dissolves in other oils but not in water. A source of energy and a building block of cells.

Fatty acids   The scientific term for fats, which are part of a group of substances called lipids. Fatty acids come in different lengths from 6-carbon to 26-carbon chains.

Fiber   Parts of plant foods that are indigestible or very slowly digested, having little effect on blood-glucose and insulin levels; sometimes called roughage.

^{18}F-2-fluoro-2-deoxyglucose   A glucose analog positron-emitting drug that is injected into the body to use as a radioactive marker for cancer cells. Cancer cells take up glucose in greater amounts, and the radioactive isotope in the drug then shows up on a PET scan, marking the location of the cancer.

Free radicals   Chemically unstable molecules that "steal" electrons from surrounding molecules. They are in the environment and naturally produced by our bodies. Excess free radicals can damage cells through oxidative activity. Think of what rust does to steel.

Fructose   A simple sugar found naturally in fruits and plants. It is also found in commercial sweeteners such as high-fructose corn syrup and crystalline fructose. Excess intake of fructose has been implicated in many health issues.

GERD   Gastrointestinal-Esophageal Reflux Disease. A medical term for severe heartburn.

Gluconeogenesis   The process by which glucose is formed in the liver from a non-carbohydrate source when blood glucose is low.

Glucose   A simple sugar. Also see blood glucose.

Glucose-avid   A term used to indicate cancers that display a preference for absorbing large amounts of blood glucose.

Glutamine   A conditionally essential amino acid that has a role in various metabolic processes. One of those roles is to provide energy to the cell in the absence of glucose. Hence, intake should be limited on a ketogenic diet for cancer individuals.

Glycerol   The "backbone" of a fatty acid or triglyceride. Imagine a capital E. The glycerol molecule represents the vertical spine of the E with fatty acids making up the horizontal lines of the E.

Glycogen   The storage form of carbohydrate in the body.

Glycolysis   The pathway by which glucose is broken down into two molecules of pyruvic acid with the generation of energy in the form of ATP.

HDL cholesterol   High-density lipoprotein; the "good" type of cholesterol.

Hydrogenated oils Vegetable oils processed to make them solid and improve their shelf life. See trans fats.

Hypertension High blood pressure.

IGF-1 The abbreviation for a protein called insulin-like growth factor 1. IGF-1 is a hormone that stimulates cellular proliferation. Studies have shown that increased levels of IGF-1 lead to increased growth of existing cancer cells.

Inflammation Part of the body's delicately balanced natural defense system against potentially damaging substances. Excessive inflammation is associated with increased risk of heart attack, stroke, diabetes, and some forms of cancer.

Insulin A hormone produced by the pancreas that signals cells to remove glucose and amino acids from the bloodstream and stop the release of fat from fat cells.

Insulin resistance A metabolic condition in which chronically high levels of circulating insulin result in body cells being desensitized and no longer able to respond properly to the insulin signals.

KD Ketogenic diet

Ketoacidosis The uncontrolled overproduction of ketones characteristic of untreated type 1 diabetes, with ketones typically five to ten times higher than in nutritional ketosis.

Ketogenesis The metabolic process in which the liver creates ketone bodies from the breakdown of fatty acids. The ketone bodies can then be metabolized within the cell mitochondria to fuel the body.

Ketogenic diet A high-fat, moderate-protein, low-carbohydrate diet used to treat various illnesses and improve health.

Ketones (ketone bodies) Substances produced by the liver from fat during accelerated fat breakdown that serve as a valuable energy source for cells throughout the body.

Ketosis A moderate and controlled level of ketones in the bloodstream that allows the body to function well with little dietary carbohydrate; also called nutritional ketosis.

Lactose The simple sugar (carbohydrate) found in milk and in milk products such as cheese and yogurt. It has a pronounced effect on insulin.

LDL cholesterol Low-density lipoprotein. Commonly known as the "bad" type of cholesterol.

Lean body mass (LBM) Body mass minus fat tissue; includes muscle, bone, organs, and connective tissue.

Legumes Most members of the bean and pea families, including lentils, chickpeas, soybeans, and peas.

Lipids A group of naturally occurring molecules that include fats, waxes, sterols such as cholesterol, fat-soluble vitamins (such as vitamins A, D, E, and K), monoglycerides, diglycerides, triglycerides, phospholipids, and others. The main biological functions of lipids include energy storage, signaling, and acting as structural components of cell membranes.

Macronutrients The three main nutrients types (fat, protein, and carbohydrate) that are the dietary sources of calories and micronutrients.

MCTs Medium-chain triglycerides. MCTs are absorbed rapidly from the intestine. In addition, MCTs do not require intestinal bile salts for digestion. Individuals who have malnutrition or digestive absorption issues are treated with MCTs because they don't require energy for absorption and utilization in the body, and they increase ketone production.

Metabolic syndrome   A group of conditions, including hypertension, high triglycerides, low HDL cholesterol, blood-glucose and insulin levels that are higher than normal, and weight carried in the middle of the body. Also known as syndrome X or insulin resistance syndrome, it predisposes one to various diseases.

Metabolism   The complex chemical processes that convert food into energy or the body's building blocks, which, in turn, become part of organs, tissues, and cells.

mg/dl   Milligrams per deciliter. A unit of measure that shows the concentration of a substance in a specific amount of fluid. It is used as a standard measurement of blood glucose in tests.

Mitochondria   Cell organelles; called the "cellular power plants" because they generate most of the cell's supply of adenosine triphosphate (ATP), the main form of cellular energy.

mM or mmol/L   Millimolar. A unit of measurement that represents a concentration of one thousandth of a solute mole per liter. Ketone levels in blood can be measured and reported in mM.

Monounsaturated fat   A type of dietary fat typically found in foods such as olive oil, canola oil, nuts, and avocados; it is also found in beef steak.

MSG   Monosodium glutamate. A chemical used to heighten taste sensations in processed foods. MSG is a neurotoxin and should be avoided on a ketogenic diet because it contains glutamate, a derivate of glutamine.

Net carbs   The carbohydrates in a food that impact your blood glucose, calculated by subtracting fiber grams in the food from total grams.

Nutrient   A chemical that an organism needs to live and grow. Nutrients are used to build and repair tissues and regulate body processes and are converted to and used as energy. For humans, fats, proteins, carbohydrates, vitamins, minerals and water are the main nutrients needed for optimal health.

Omega-3 fatty acids   A group of essential polyunsaturated fats found in green algae, cold-water fish, fish oil, flaxseed oil, and some other nut and vegetable oils. Omega-3 fatty acids have an anti-inflammatory effect on body systems.

Omega-6 fatty acids   A group of essential polyunsaturated fats found in many vegetable oils and also in meats from animals fed corn, soybeans, and certain other vegetable products. Omega-6 fatty acids have an inflammatory downstream effect on body systems.

Oxidative stress   The condition in which the production of reactive oxygen species (ROS) through various metabolic pathways is at a greater rate than the body's defense system of antioxidants can handle, resulting in cellular damage at the molecular level. Oxidative stress is thought to play a part in many disease processes.

Partially hydrogenated oil   Oil that has been solidified using a catalytic chemical manufacturing process. See trans fats.

PET scan   A nuclear medicine imaging technique that produces a three-dimensional image or picture of functional processes in the body. The system detects radiation emitted indirectly by a positron-emitting tracer, which is introduced into the body on a biologically active molecule.

Plaque   A buildup in the arteries of cholesterol, fat, calcium, and other substances that can block blood flow, which can result in a heart attack or stroke.

Polyunsaturated fats   Fats with a chemical structure that keeps them liquid at cold temperatures; oils from corn, soybean, sunflower, safflower, cottonseed, grape seed, flaxseed, sesame seed, some nuts, and fatty fish are typically high in polyunsaturated fat.

Pre-diabetes   A condition in which blood-glucose levels are higher than normal but fall short of full-blown diabetes.

Protein   One of the three macronutrients found in food; used for energy and building blocks of cells. Proteins are made up of chains of amino acids.

Radiation therapy   The medical use of targeted ionizing radiation as part of cancer treatment to control or kill malignant cells through damaging the cell DNA.

RDA   Recommended daily allowance. The average daily dietary intake level of a nutrient that is sufficient to meet the nutrient requirements of nearly all (approximately 98%) healthy individuals.

Resistance exercise   Any exercise that builds muscle strength; also called weight-bearing or anaerobic exercise.

Satiety   A pleasurable sense of fullness.

Saturated fats   Fats that are solid at room temperature; the majority of fat in butter, lard, suet, palm and coconut oil.

Substrate   In chemistry, a substance that is acted upon in a biochemical reaction.

Sucrose   Table sugar. Sucrose is composed of two monosaccharides or simple sugars called glucose and fructose.

Sugar alcohols   Sweeteners such as glycerin, mannitol, erythritol, sorbitol, and xylitol that have little or no impact on most people's blood glucose. They are, however, anti-ketogenic in that they interfere with ketosis.

Trans fats   Fats found in partially hydrogenated or hydrogenated vegetable oil; typically used in fried foods, baked goods, and other products. A high intake of trans fats is associated with increased heart-attack risk.

Triglycerides   The major form of fat that circulates in the bloodstream and is stored as body fat. High levels are associated with a greater risk of heart disease. A high-carb diet increases triglycerides.

Type 1 diabetes   An autoimmune disease in which the cells that secrete insulin in the pancreas have been damaged or destroyed. The result is that the body is unable to make insulin, and without insulin, the body cannot move glucose from the bloodstream into the cells. As a result, the sugar levels in the blood become very high, and this high blood glucose damages the body systems. If not treated by insulin injections, type 1 diabetics can develop serious health problems such as blindness, kidney disease, heart disease, and nerve damage.

Type 2 diabetes   By far the more common type of diabetes; it is the type mostly strongly associated with insulin resistance. It is the most common health result of chronically elevated blood-glucose and insulin levels. These elevated levels of sugar and insulin have the effect of "numbing" the cellular processes that are involved with moving sugar from the bloodstream to the cells. In other words, the cells cannot "hear" the insulin asking to move sugar into the cells. As a result, the body cannot respond to the insulin requests to move blood glucose into the cells, and the sugar in the bloodstream rises to damaging levels.

Unsaturated fat   Monounsaturated fats (such as olive oil) and polyunsaturated fats (found in most vegetable and fish oils). They are usually liquid at room temperature.

Endnotes

1 Warburg OH. The classic: The chemical constitution of respiration ferment. *Clin Orthop Relat Res.* 2010 Nov;468(11): 2833–9. Reprint.

2 Brand RA. Biographical Sketch: Otto Heinrich Warburg, PhD, MD. *Clin Orthop Relat Res.* 2010;468(11):2831–2832.

3 Seyfried, Thomas N. *Cancer as a Metabolic Disease: On the Origin, Management, and Prevention of Cancer.* Hoboken: John Wiley & Sons, 2012.

4 Paoli A, Rubini A, Volek JS, Grimaldi KA. *Eur J Clin Nutr.* 2013 Aug;67(8):789-96. Review. Erratum in: *Eur J Clin Nutr.* 2014 May;68(5):641.

5 Scott EM, Greenwood JP, Vacca G, Stoker JB, Gilbey SG, Mary DA. Carbohydrate ingestion, with transient endogenous insulinaemia, produces both sympathetic activation and vasodilatation in normal humans. *Clin Sci (Lond).* 2002 May;102(5): 523–9.

6 Masino, SA, ed. *Ketogenic Diet and Metabolic Therapies: Expanded Roles in Health and Disease.* Chapter 12. Oxford: Oxford University Press, 2017.

7 Mukherjee P, Sotnikov AV, Mangian HJ, Zhou JR, Visek WJ, Clinton SK. Energy intake and prostate tumor growth, angiogenesis, and vascular endothelial growth factor expression. *J Natl Cancer Inst.* 1999;91:512–523.

8 Poff AM, Ward N, Seyfried TN, Arnold P, D'Agostino DP. Non-Toxic Metabolic Management of Metastatic Cancer in VM Mice: Novel Combination of Ketogenic Diet, Ketone Supplementation, and Hyperbaric Oxygen Therapy. *PLoS One.* 2015 Jun 10;10(6):e0127407.

9 Lardy HA, Phillips PH. 1945. Studies of fat and carbohydrate oxidation in mammalian spermatozoa. *Arch. Biochem.* 6:53–61

10 Veech R. L. (2004) The therapeutic implications of ketone bodies: The effects of ketone bodies in pathological conditions: Ketosis, ketogenic diet, redox states, insulin resistance, and mitochondrial metabolism. *Prostaglandins, Leukotrienes, and Essential Fatty Acids* 70: 309–319.

11 Godsland IF. Insulin resistance and hyperinsulinaemia in the development and progression of cancer. *Clinical Science* (London, England : 1979). 2009;118(Pt 5):315-332.

12 Braun S, Bitton-Worms K, LeRoith D. The Link between the Metabolic Syndrome and Cancer. *International Journal of Biological Sciences.* 2011;7(7):1003-1015.

13 Stafford P, Abdelwahab MG, Kim DY, Preul MC, Rho JM, Scheck AC. The ketogenic diet reverses gene expression patterns and reduces reactive oxygen species levels when used as an adjuvant therapy for glioma. *Nutr Metab (Lond).* 2010 Sep 10;7:74

14 Abdelwahab MG, Fenton KE, Preul MC, et al. The Ketogenic Diet Is an Effective Adjuvant to Radiation Therapy for the Treatment of Malignant Glioma. Canoll P, ed. *PLoS ONE.* 2012;7(5):e36197. Nebeling LC, Miraldi F, Shurin SB, Lerner E. Effects of a ketogenic diet on tumor metabolism and nutritional status in pediatric oncology patients: two case reports. *J Am Coll Nutr.* 1995 Apr;14(2):202.

15 Newman JC, Verdin E. Ketone bodies as signaling metabolites. *Trends Endocrinol Metab.* 2014 Jan;25(1): 42–52. Epub 2013 Oct 18. Review.

16 Nebeling LC, Miraldi F, Shurin SB, Lerner E. Effects of a ketogenic diet on tumor metabolism and nutritional status in pediatric oncology patients: two case reports. *J Am Coll Nutr.* 1995 Apr;14(2):202. Available at http://www.ncbi.nlm.nih.gov/pubmed/7790697.

17 Fine EJ, Segal-Isaacson CJ, Feinman RD, Herszkopf S, Romano MC, Tomuta N, Bontempo AF, Negassa A, Sparano JA. Targeting insulin inhibition as a metabolic therapy in advanced cancer: a pilot safety and feasibility dietary trial in 10 patients. *Nutrition.* 2012 Oct;28(10):1028-35.

18 Abdelwahab MG, Fenton KE, Preul MC, et al. The Ketogenic Diet Is an Effective Adjuvant to Radiation Therapy for the Treatment of Malignant Glioma. Canoll P, ed. *PLoS ONE.* 2012;7(5):e36197.

19 Schmidt M, Pfetzer N, Schwab M, Strauss I, Kämmerer U. Effects of a ketogenic diet on the quality of life in 16 patients with advanced cancer: A pilot trial. *Nutrition & Metabolism.* 2011;8:54. doi:10.1186/1743-7075-8-54.

20 Seyfried TN, Shelton LM. Cancer as a metabolic disease. *Nutr Metab (Lond).* 2010 Jan 27;7:7.

21 Seyfried TN, Sanderson TM, El-Abbadi MM, McGowan R, Mukherjee P. Role of glucose and ketone bodies in the metabolic control of experimental brain cancer. *Br J Cancer.* 2003 Oct 6;89(7):1375–82.

22 Mulrooney TJ, Marsh J, Urits I, Seyfried TN, Mukherjee P. Influence of caloric restriction on constitutive expression of NF-κB in an experimental mouse astrocytoma. *PLoS One.* 2011 Mar 30;6(3):e18085.

23 Seyfried TN, Shelton LM. Cancer as a metabolic disease. *Nutr Metab (Lond).* 2010 Jan 27;7:7.

24 Scheck AC, Abdelwahab MG, Fenton KE, Stafford P. The ketogenic diet for the treatment of glioma: insights from genetic profiling. *Epilepsy Res.* 2012 Jul;100(3):327–37.

25 Stafford P, Abdelwahab MG, Kim DY, Preul MC, Rho JM, Scheck AC. The ketogenic diet reverses gene expression patterns and reduces reactive oxygen species levels when used as an adjuvant therapy for glioma. *Nutr Metab (Lond).* 2010 Sep 10;7:74.

26 Klement RJ, Sweeney RA. Impact of a ketogenic diet intervention during radiotherapy on body composition: I. Initial clinical experience with six prospectively studied patients. *BMC Res Notes.* 2016 Mar 5;9:143.

27 Jansen N, Walach H. The development of tumours under a ketogenic diet in association with the novel tumour marker TKTL1: A case series in general practice. *Oncol Lett.* 2016 Jan;11(1):584–592.

28 Klement RJ, Champ CE, Otto C, Kämmerer U. Anti-Tumor Effects of Ketogenic Diets in Mice: A Meta-Analysis. *PLoS One.* 2016 May 9;11(5):e0155050.

29 Stafford P, Abdelwahab MG, Kim DY, Preul MC, Rho JM, Scheck AC. The ketogenic diet reverses gene expression patterns and reduces reactive oxygen species levels when used as an adjuvant therapy for glioma. *Nutr Metab (Lond).* 2010 Sep 10;7:74.

30 Lussier DM, Woolf EC, Johnson JL, Brooks KS, Blattman JN, Scheck AC. Enhanced immunity in a mouse model of malignant glioma is mediated by a therapeutic ketogenic diet. *BMC Cancer.* 2016 May 13;16:310.

31 D'Agostino DP, Pilla R, Held HE, Landon CS, Puchowicz M, Brunengraber H, Ari C, Arnold P, Dean JB. Therapeutic ketosis with ketone ester delays central nervous system oxygen toxicity seizures in rats. *Am J Physiol Regul Integr Comp Physiol.* 2013 May 15;304(10):R829-36.

32 The Use Of Ketone Esters For Prevention Of Cns Oxygen Toxicity Patent application available at http://www.freepatentsonline.com/WO2012154837A2.html.

33 Poff A, Ward N, Seyfried T, D'Agostino D. Combination ketogenic diet, ketone supplementation, and hyperbaric oxygen therapy inhibits metastatic spread, slows tumor growth, and increases survival time in mice with metastatic cancer. *The FASEB Journal.* April 2014,vol. 28 no. 1 Supplement 123.7.

34 Semenza GL. Regulation of cancer cell metabolism by hypoxia-inducible factor 1. *Semin Cancer Biol.* 2009 Feb;19(1):12–6.

35 Yang SL, Ren QG, Wen L, Hu JL. Clinicopathological and prognostic significance of hypoxia-inducible factor-1 alpha in lung cancer: a systematic review with meta-analysis. *J Huazhong Univ Sci Technolog Med Sci.* 2016 Jun;36(3):321–7.

36 Zhang D, Cui L, Li SS, Wang F. Insulin and hypoxia-inducible factor-1 cooperate in pancreatic cancer cells to increase cell viability. *Oncol Lett.* 2015 Sep;10(3):1545–1550. Epub 2015 Jun 17.

37 Poff AM, Ward N, Seyfried TN, Arnold P, D'Agostino DP. Non-Toxic Metabolic Management of Metastatic Cancer in VM Mice: Novel Combination of Ketogenic Diet, Ketone Supplementation, and Hyperbaric Oxygen Therapy. *PLoS One.* 2015 Jun 10;10(6):e0127407.

38 Poff AM, Ari C, Seyfried TN, D'Agostino DP. The ketogenic diet and hyperbaric oxygen therapy prolong survival in mice with systemic metastatic cancer. *PLoS One.* 2013 Jun 5;8(6):e65522.

39 University of South Florida Health Sciences. Available at https: //hscweb3.hsc.usf.edu/blog/2015/06/10/usf-researchers-develop-novel-ketone-supplements-to-enhance-non-toxic-cancer-therapy/.

40 Woolf EC, Scheck AC. The ketogenic diet for the treatment of malignant glioma. *Journal of Lipid Research.* 2015;56(1):5-10.

41 National Cancer Institute. *Metformin: Can a Diabetes Drug Help Prevent Cancer?* Available at http://www.cancer.gov/about-cancer/causes-prevention/research/metformin.

42 Bonnet S, Archer SL, Allalunis-Turner J, Haromy A, Beaulieu C, Thompson R, et al. A mitochondria-K+ channel axis is suppressed in cancer and its normalization promotes apoptosis and inhibits cancer growth. *Cancer Cell.* 2007 Jan;11(1):37–51.

43 Kaufmann P, Engelstad K, Wei Y, Jhung S, Sano MC, Shungu DC, Millar WS, Hong X, Gooch CL, Mao X, Pascual JM, Hirano M, Stacpoole PW, DiMauro S, De Vivo DC. Dichloroacetate causes toxic neuropathy in MELAS: a randomized, controlled clini-cal trial. *Neurology.* 2006 Feb 14;66(3):324-30.

44 Azemar M, Hildenbrand B, Haering B, Heim ME, Unger C. Clinical benefit in patients with advanced solid tumors treated with modified citrus pectin: a prospective pilot study. *Clin Med Oncol.* 2007;1: 73–80.

45 Ramachandran C, Wilk BJ, Hotchkiss A, Chau H, Eliaz I, Melnick SJ. Activation of human T-helper/inducer cell, T-cytotoxic cell, B-cell, and natural killer (NK)-cells and induction of natural killer cell activity against K562 chronic myeloid leukemia cells with modified citrus pectin. *BMC Complement Altern Med.* 2011 Aug 4;11:59.

46 Reishi Mushroom. Memorial Sloan Kettering Cancer Center Integrative Medicine. Available at https://www.mskcc.org/cancer-care/integrative-medicine/herbs/reishi-mushroom. Accessed January 8, 2017.

47 Meidenbauer JJ, Mukherjee P, Seyfried TN. The glucose ketone index calculator: a simple tool to monitor therapeutic efficacy for metabolic management of brain cancer. *Nutr Metab (Lond).* 2015;12(1):12.

48 Shukla SK, Gebregiworgis T, Purohit V, Chaika NV, Gunda V, Radhakrishnan P, Mehla K, Pipinos II, Powers R, Yu F, Singh PK. Metabolic reprogramming induced by ketone bodies diminishes pancreatic cancer cachexia. *Cancer Metab.* 2014 Sep 1;2:18.

49 Rosedale, Ron. Cholesterol is NOT the cause of heart disease. Available at http://drrosedale.com/Cholesterol_is_NOT_the_cause_of_heart_disease.htm#ixzz4H35CzptL

50 Tennyson C, Lee R, Attia R. Is there a role for HbA1c in predicting mortality and morbidity outcomes after coronary artery bypass graft surgery? *Interact Cardiovasc Thorac Surg.* 2013 Dec;17(6): 1000-8. Epub 2013 Sep 10. Review.

51 Straub RH. Insulin resistance, selfish brain, and selfish immune system: an evolutionarily positively selected program used in chronic inflammatory diseases. *Arthritis Research & Therapy.* 2014;16(Suppl 2):S4.

52 Samaha FF, Foster GD, Makris AP. Low-carbohydrate diets, obesity, and metabolic risk factors for cardiovascular disease. *Curr Atheroscler Rep.* 2007 Dec;9(6): 441-7. Review.

53 Dashti HM, Mathew TC, Khadada M, Al-Mousawi M, Talib H, Asfar SK, Behbahani AI, Al-Zaid NS. Beneficial effects of ketogenic diet in obese diabetic subjects. *Mol Cell Biochem.* 2007 Aug;302(1-2):249-56.

54 Samaha FF, Foster GD, Makris AP. Low-carbohydrate diets, obesity, and metabolic risk factors for cardiovascular disease. *Curr Atheroscler Rep.* 2007 Dec;9(6): 441-7. Review.

55 Feinman RD, Pogozelski WK, Astrup A, Bernstein RK, Fine EJ, Westman EC, et al. Dietary carbohydrate restriction as the first approach in diabetes management: critical review and evidence base. *Nutrition.* 2015 Jan;31(1):1-13.

56 Westman EC, Yancy WS Jr, Mavropoulos JC, Marquart M, McDuffie JR. The effect of a low-carbohydrate, ketogenic diet versus a low-glycemic index diet on glycemic control in type 2 diabetes mellitus. *Nutr Metab (Lond).* 2008 Dec 19;5:36.

57 Nielsen JV, Gando C, Joensson E, Paulsson C. Low carbohydrate diet in type 1 diabetes, long-term improvement and adherence: A clinical audit. *Diabetol Metab Syndr.* 2012 May 31;4(1):23.

58 Manrique C, Lastra G, Sowers JR. New insights into insulin action and resistance in the vasculature. *Annals of the New York Academy of Sciences.* 2014;1311(1):138-150.

59 Forsythe CE, Phinney SD, Fernandez ML, Quann EE, Wood RJ, Bibus DM, Kraemer WJ, Feinman RD, Volek JS. Comparison of low fat and low carbohydrate diets on circulating fatty acid composition and markers of inflammation. *Lipids.* 2008 Jan;43(1):65-77.

60 Nachman F, Vázquez H, González A, Andrenacci P, Compagni L, Reyes H, Sugai E, Moreno ML, Smecuol E, Hwang HJ, Sánchez IP, Mauriño E, Bai JC. Gastroesophageal reflux symptoms in patients with celiac disease and the effects of a gluten-free diet. *Clin Gastroenterol Hepatol.* 2011 Mar;9(3):214-9.

61 Austin GL, Thiny MT, Westman EC, Yancy WS Jr, Shaheen NJ. A very low-carbohydrate diet improves gastroesophageal reflux and its symptoms. *Dig Dis Sci.* 2006 Aug;51(8):1307-12.

62 Struzycka I. The oral microbiome in dental caries. *Pol J Microbiol.* 2014;63(2):127-35. Review.

63 Demmer RT, Jacobs DR Jr, Singh R, Zuk A, Rosenbaum M, Papapanou PN, Desvarieux M. Periodontal Bacteria and Prediabetes Prevalence in ORIGINS: The Oral Infections, Glucose Intolerance, and Insulin Resistance Study. *J Dent Res.* 2015 Sep;94(9 Suppl):201S-11S.

64 Phelps JR, Siemers SV, El-Mallakh RS. The ketogenic diet for type II bipolar disorder. *Neurocase.* 2013;19(5):423-6.

65 Kraft BD, Westman EC. Schizophrenia, gluten, and low-carbohydrate, ketogenic diets: a case report and review of the literature. *Nutr Metab (Lond).* 2009 Feb 26;6:10.

66 Giovannucci E. Metabolic syndrome, hyperinsulinemia, and colon cancer: a review. *Am J Clin Nutr.* 2007 Sep;86(3):s836-42. Review.

67 Parekh N, Lin Y, Hayes RB, Albu JB, Lu-Yao GL. Longitudinal associations of blood markers of insulin and glucose concentrations and cancer mortality in the Third National Health and Nutrition Examination Survey. Cancer causes & control : CCC. 2010;21(4):10.1007/s10552-009-9492-y.

68 Seyfried TN, Flores RE, Poff AM, D'Agostino DP. Cancer as a metabolic disease: implications for novel therapeutics. *Carcinogenesis.* 2014 Mar;35(3):515-27. Review.

69 Gibson AA, Seimon RV, Lee CM, Ayre J, Franklin J, Markovic TP, Caterson ID, Sainsbury A. Do ketogenic diets really suppress appetite? A systematic review and meta-analysis. *Obes Rev.* 2015 Jan;16(1):64-76. Review.

70 Westman EC, Yancy WS, Edman JS, Tomlin KF, Perkins CE. Effect of 6-month adherence to a very low carbohydrate diet program. *Am J Med.* 2002 Jul;113(1):30-6.

71 Brehm BJ, Seeley RJ, Daniels SR, D'Alessio DA. A randomized trial comparing a very low carbohydrate diet and a calorie-restricted low fat diet on body weight and cardiovascular risk factors in healthy women. *J Clin Endocrinol Metab.* 2003 Apr;88(4):1617-23.

72 Paoli A, Rubini A, Volek JS, Grimaldi KA. Beyond weight loss: a review of the therapeutic uses of very-low-carbohydrate (ketogenic) diets. *Eur J Clin Nutr.* 2013 Aug;67(8):789-96. Review. Erratum in: *Eur J Clin Nutr.* 2014 May;68(5):641.

73 Stafstrom CE, Rho JM. The ketogenic diet as a treatment paradigm for diverse neurological disorders. *Front Pharmacol.* 2012 Apr 9;3:59.

74 Davis E. *Checking Blood Sugar.* Ketogenic Diet Resource website. Available at http: //www.ketogenic-diet-resource.com/checking-blood-sugar.html

75 USDA Food Composition Database. Available at http://ndb.nal.usda.gov/.

76 Hartmann S, Larkus M, Steinhart H. (1998). Natural occurrence of steroid hormones in food. *Food Chemistry,* 62 (1): 7–20. Available at http://www.ketogenic-diet-resource.com/support-files/natural_occurrence_of_steroid_hormones_in_food.pdf.

77 Thorning TK, Raben A, Tholstrup T, Soedamah-Muthu SS, Givens I, Astrup A. Milk and dairy products: good or bad for human health? An assessment of the totality of scientific evidence. *Food Nutr Res.* 2016 Nov 22;60:32527.

78 Charlie Foundation. Available at http://www.charliefoundation.org/resources-tools/resources-3/low-carb.

79 People who have not progressed to advanced stages of cancer, are not physically weak and are not underweight or losing weight due to the effects of medical treatments.

80 *Calculate Your Body Mass Index.* National Heart, Lung and Blood Institute. Available at http://www.nhlbi.nih.gov/guidelines/obesity/BMI/bmicalc.htm

81 *Intermittent Fasting.* Wikipedia Available at http://en.wikipedia.org/wiki/Intermittent_fasting

82 Davis, Ellen. *Gluconeogenesis.* Available at http://www.ketogenic-diet-resource.com/gluconeogenesis.html

83 Zupec-Kania, Beth. *Modified Ketogenic Diet Therapy.* The Charlie Foundation for Ketogenic Diet Therapies, 2013.

84 Sayin VI, Ibrahim MX, Larsson E, Nilsson JA, Lindahl P, Bergo MO. Antioxidants accelerate lung cancer progression in mice. *Sci Transl Med.* 2014 Jan 29;6(221):221ra15.

About the Author

Ellen Davis has a Master's degree in Applied Clinical Nutrition from New York Chiropractic College. She created Ketogenic-Diet-Resource.com, a website showcasing the research on the positive health effects of ketogenic diets and has written articles about ketogenic diets for Well Being Journal, Terry's Naturally magazine and Healthy Living magazine.

In addition to *Fight Cancer with a Ketogenic Diet*, Ellen has authored several other books, including *Conquer Type 2 Diabetes with a Ketogenic Diet* and *The Ketogenic Diet for Type 1 Diabetes*, both written with her coauthor, Keith Runyan, MD, a physician who manages his type 1 diabetes successfully with a ketogenic diet. Her latest book, *The Ketone Cure*, will be published in 2017.

Visit

ketogenic-diet-resource.com

for more information about the research on and applications for ketogenic diets, and to purchase additional books by Ellen Davis:

The Ketogenic Diet for Type 1 Diabetes

Conquer Type 2 Diabetes with a Ketogenic Diet

The Ketone Cure (2017)

Made in the USA
Middletown, DE
25 July 2018